Manual of F
Leade

MW00845401

Notice

Medicine is an ever-changing science. As new research and clinical experience broaden our knowledge, changes in treatment and drug therapy are required. The author and the publisher of this work have checked with sources believed to be reliable in their efforts to provide information that is complete and generally in accord with the standards accepted at the time of publication. However, in view of the possibility of human error or changes in medical sciences, neither the author nor the publisher nor any other party who has been involved in the preparation or publication of this work warrants that the information contained herein is in every respect accurate or complete, and they disclaim all responsibility for any errors or omissions or for the results obtained from use of the information contained in this work. Readers are encouraged to confirm the information contained herein with other sources. For example and in particular, readers are advised to check the product information sheet included in the package of each drug they plan to administer to be certain that the information contained in this work is accurate and that changes have not been made in the recommended dose or in the contraindications for administration. This recommendation is of particular importance in connection with new or infrequently used drugs.

Manual of Healthcare Leadership:
Essential Strategies for Physician and Administrative Leaders

Donald N. Lombardi, PhD, USMC(R)
Alexander Crombie Humphreys Distinguished Associate Professor
Director, Stevens Healthcare Educational Partnership
Academic Director, Stevens Veterans Office
Hoboken, New Jersey

Anthony D. Slonim, MD, DrPH
Executive Vice President/Chief Medical Officer
Barnabas Health
West Orange, New Jersey
Professor, Medicine, Pediatrics, Community and Public Health
University of Medicine and Dentistry of New Jersey
New Jersey Medical School
Newark, New Jersey

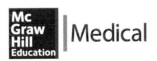

New York   Chicago   San Francisco   Athens   London   Madrid
Mexico City   Milan   New Delhi   Singapore   Sydney   Toronto

Manual of Healthcare Leadership: Essential Strategies for Physician and Administrative Leaders

1 2 3 4 5 6 7 8 9 0   MPM   28 27 26 25 24

ISBN 978-0-07-179484-8
MHID 0-07-179484-0

This book was set in Times by Cenveo® Publisher Services.
The editors were James F. Shanahan and Kim J. Davis.
The production supervisor was Richard Ruzycka.
Project management was provided by Anupriya Tyagi of Cenveo Publisher Services.
Markono Print Media Pte Ltd was printer and binder.
This book is printed on acid-free paper.
Library of Congress Cataloging-in-Publication Data

This book is printed on acid-free paper.

Library of Congress Cataloging-in-Publication Data

Lombardi, Donald N., 1956-
    Manual of healthcare leadership: essential strategies for physician and administrative leaders/Donald N. Lombardi, Anthony D. Slonim.
        p. cm.
    Includes index.
    ISBN-13: 978-0-07-179484-8 (pbk.: alk. paper)
    ISBN-10: 0-07-179484-0 (pbk.: alk. paper)   1. Health services administration.
    2. Health facilities—Personnel management.   3. Leadership.   I. Slonim, Anthony D.
    II. Title.
    RA971.35.L655   2014
    362.1068'4—dc23
                                                                        2013036287

The authors dedicate this book to
Deborah Ann, Samantha, and Michael.

Contents

CHAPTER SIX

Motivation, Communication, and Negotiation...... 167

CHAPTER SEVEN

Maximizing Team Action and Individual Performance.. 209

Preface

"It is a riddle, wrapped in a mystery, inside an enigma; but perhaps there is a key." These words, spoken in 1939 by Winston Churchill, were focused on the changing global environment with its attendant looming change and crisis. However, this quote could be relevant to both the current condition of health care and the intent of this book to provide a key. As another quote—**doing more with less**—transforms into **doing everything with nothing**, health care is experiencing change, crisis, and challenge at an unprecedented level. A phalanx of puzzling new laws and regulations are making reimbursement and other pathways to profit for the majority of healthcare organizations—most of which are nonprofit—vexing and perilous, threatening the very existence and solvency of these selfless, community-driven organizations. The patient, heretofore considered a constituent who had unconditional abiding trust in his or her doctor and local healthcare organization, has now become jaded due to the media and political complexes making health care more complex in popular perception. As trust erodes, the patient has become a skeptical and wary customer attached to the mantra **consumer beware!**

As these new and potentially nefarious external forces impel change on the healthcare organization, internal reactions lead to more strife and a need for rebounding clarity. While operating budgets shrink, healthcare leaders have to become more resourceful in their utilization of precious resources from allocated staff to allocated financial assets. As demand for new and improved services resonates from the media to the customer/patient and then land with a thud on the local healthcare organization, healthcare leaders must ensure that their sector of the organization is not only providing vanguard, cutting-edge services but is providing those services at a high-quality level, lest patient satisfaction scores and other demanding assessments fall into the negative column. And as steady staff members become unsteadied and unsure in undertaking their daily job responsibilities in the face of all of this change, which they firmly believe will get worse before it gets better, the healthcare and physician leaders in our profession must be beacons of hope, stewards of a purposeful course, and a source of positive impact and progressive growth and development—all in one day, every day. A tough charter indeed and one that we hope can be met with this book.

The Manual of Healthcare Leadership: Essential Strategies for Healthcare and Physician Leaders is intended to be an immediately useful, ready-to-apply handbook as you undertake this tough charter. We are fortunate as authors to have garnered a practical perspective based on over 60 years of combined experience in healthcare, physician, and organizational leadership. We also have the opportunity to be both innovators and educators at several leading healthcare and medical institutions, and our work has included curriculum design and course content. We have been provided with a wealth of acumen gleaned from the most important source of effective healthcare and physician leadership strategy: the knowledge and practices of hundreds of successful healthcare and physician leaders at all decision-making levels in scores of healthcare organizations that have provided their communities with stellar health care based on the true power of people.

Rather than providing another theoretic tome or a catchy collection of trendy psychobabble phrases and vacuous argot, this book seeks to provide relevant and resonant information by using a very accessible and viable two-part cadence. In each chapter, first an overall aegis of information and insight into critical leadership and management accountability is provided based on current practice and effective employ. Second, detailed but efficiently presented information is augmented by strategies and practical applications that can be employed by your organization immediately upon reading and understanding their import and employ. A reader can certainly start on page one of this book and continue apace to the last page, all the while acquiring useful and applicable knowledge, as we have organized the content in a sequence that not only charts the initial responsibilities of a healthcare leader, but also parallels the chronology of management and leadership development in a progressive manner. Additionally, each chapter contains specific leadership and management responsibility that can be accessed as needed due to the clarity of enumerated organization and the **ready-to-use** proven strategy resources provided.

Our intention for this book—in fact, our sincerest aspiration for this effort—is that all our readers will find immediate use which will help them navigate the most potentially treacherous aspects of their job—**maximizing the performance of each staff member in the interest of collectively providing peerless health care to their service community**. In this regard, readers of this book can range from senior executives to board members to department heads to team leaders and supervisors to students, both in the classroom and on the job, who aspire to become leaders in the most demanding of all human services—healthcare and medical leadership. As patients are increasingly aware of costs and new dimensions of the medical services, they feel compelled to closely scrutinize every aspect of health care delivery. Accordingly, sharp assessments are conducted in every stage in the delivery of the health care that seems to be both more expensive and more complex. And while they might not be experts in medical services nor health care delivery economics, current patients do consider themselves very well qualified to make a critical assessment on the quality of compassion and communication extended to them in the care process. The human touch must be extended by each and every member of a healthcare organization and encouraged by the healthcare leader who is charged with the critical responsibility of selecting, training, guiding, and assessing members of their staff. While undertaking this responsibility, the healthcare leader must also negotiate, plan, resolve problems, manage change and crisis, and handle any other challenges that require a near Herculean effort on a daily basis.

This book will be a capable resource in assisting you in undertaking these somewhat daunting responsibilities. Each segment of the book presents the why, what, and how of each critical management and leadership responsibility. That is, the book provides exposition of the rationale and need for a specific management and leadership responsibility, explains the context for the aspect of management, and then provides specific strategies and proven systems in such critical areas as selecting the right staff member, conducting a criterion-based performance evaluation, and preparing change action plan for your team. Instruction is provided in this book not only with text, but each diagram and resource section has been innovated purposefully to specifically provide sequential thinking and progressive application for a critical dimension of management and leadership. Honoring the Druckerian Philosophy that **management** involves **doing things right,** and **leadership** is all about **doing the right things,** a plethora of strategies throughout the text are presented with the triad of why, what, and how that should be easily resonant and evidently applicable to your specific responsibilities as a healthcare manager and leader.

The book begins with strategies on how to make the vexing transition from staff member or professional to manager and leader. Chapter 1 "Making the Transition to Physician Leader" uses the platform of the Peter Principle of Healthcare to help you to avoid common pitfalls in making a smooth transition and ensuring that your initial foray into management is one teeming with positive impact and a strong foundation for success. Chapter 2 "The PACT System for Strategic Leadership Communication" continues the discourse by presenting the PACT Formula, a very intuitive application that will assist you in setting goals and plans, establishing policy, and enhancing your foundation of management and leadership. Chapter 3 "A Healthcare Leader's Guide to People Management" provides a comprehensive perspective on people management and includes specific instruction on how to manage all of your human capital. The chapter's resource section is supplemented by a validated interviewing and selection system that is in use at many leading healthcare organizations to help you select the absolute best candidate from both internal and external application pools. Chapter 4 "Dealing with Politics, Problems, and Process" deals in a forthright, direct, and thoughtful manner with the potentially perilous combination of change, crisis, and conflict. In addition to providing tutelage on the catalytic factors of this omnipresent and often treacherous confluence, a change management guide is detailed in the resource section that will assist you in being proactive in not only avoiding problems but truly turning challenges into opportunities past the clichés and bromides. Chapter 5 "Practical Strategy for Planning" delves into the essential leadership accountability of planning by examining various aspects of planning and delineating a practicum on the major steps inherent to the planning process. The chapter concludes with a very powerful tool, the Change Readiness Index (CRI), that has been maximized by a number of healthcare and medical organizations as a comparative organizational survey and scorecard that can then act as the foundation for truly meaningful and efficacious strategic planning.

In Chapter 6 "Motivation, Communication, and Negotiation," the book pivots toward the trifecta of communication, motivation, and negotiation–the individual accountabilities of a healthcare leader that can have profound positive impact on all members of the organization. The chapter's resource section contains a criterion-based performance evaluation system used by leading healthcare medical organizations which can also be implemented as it has been at many progressive organizations as a **pay**

for performance system that truly enhances positive motivation for the strong members of the organization while eliminating those who lack motivation, ability, or knowledge to contribute at a level commiserate with their paycheck. Chapter 7 "Maximizing Team Action and Individual Performance" fuses the individual responsibilities of the leader with the selfless action vital to inspiring a team with the dynamics of strong team building that ensures your staff is well positioned for both present and future demands. A maxim in health care is that **what we did today is likely not going to be good enough for tomorrow**. Chapter 8 "Encouraging Creativity and Innovation" moves to the important responsibilities of inspiring innovation and creativity by pragmatically and logically illustrating several strategies and tactical actions that can be used to tap creative contribution from both the staff members who you believe are capable of being thought leaders, as well as those who might be **hidden gems** among your charges. In a similar vein, Chapter 9 "Education and Development Strategies" helps you to prepare for tomorrow by exploring practical strategies in the areas of education and development. A very useful job resource is provided at the end of this chapter to help your leadership and management development by exploring critical questions attendant to many situations you may face on a daily basis and arriving through the use of those questions at the best possible solutions. Finally, Chapter 10 "Applying the C-Formula: Strategies for Staff Engagement" brings the book to a strong functional conclusion by detailing the critical C-Formula that provides both a comprehensive review of the critical lessons contained in this book and puts forth some more new and viable strategies for your use.

We would like to acknowledge and thank all of the great folks at McGraw-Hill Education, all of our friends and colleagues in the wonderful world of healthcare and medical management and leadership, and, most of all, our families who have been the prime teachers of our leadership acumen. We hope that the knowledge, support, inspiration, and care provided by all of these great people have helped to shape this book and that it will be useful as you continue to do good work.

Donald N. Lombardi
Anthony D. Slonim

CHAPTER ONE

Making the Transition to Healthcare and Physician Leadership

This chapter will start with identifying the biggest contrasts between physician and physician leaders. In understanding both the contrast and comparative elements of each role, you can prepare to make a progressive, positive transition into your new role as a healthcare or physician leader. We will then move to some initial practical perspectives and strategies which will help you undertake this critical transition effectively and employ this handbook as a readily useful reference for undertaking your new role.

DIFFERENCE BETWEEN PROFESSIONAL AND MANAGERIAL ROLES

Self-Direction Versus Selfless Service

As a healthcare professional, you are in a position that is more self-directed. Your job description reflects a range of activities that you pretty much control and that require mastery of some technical discipline. (Here, technical discipline includes specific medical skills, as well as acumen in accounting, information technology, customer care, and a host of other specific skills.) In your daily work, you make technical judgments without undue reliance on others, and external and internal organizational dynamics have little impact on your daily activities.

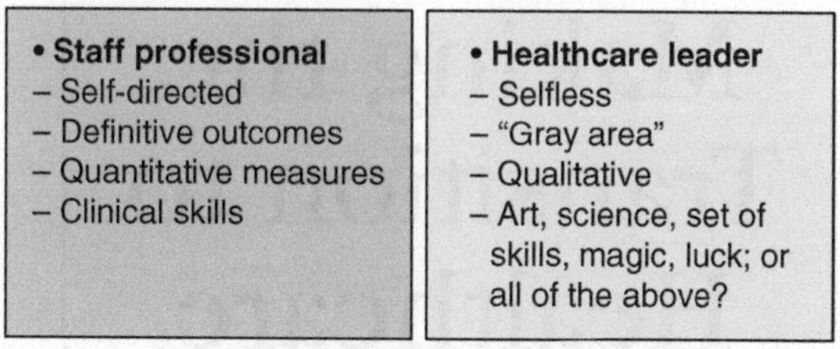

• Staff professional	• Healthcare leader
– Self-directed	– Selfless
– Definitive outcomes	– "Gray area"
– Quantitative measures	– Qualitative
– Clinical skills	– Art, science, set of skills, magic, luck; or all of the above?

FIGURE 1–1.   The Peter Principle of H/C leadership.

In essence, professionals are responsible first and foremost for their own performance: you are the key factor in determining the level of success you experience and what contribution you make to your organization.

As a physician leader, by contrast, you are in an area of selfless service (Figure 1–1), which depicts the applicable of The Peter Principle to health care. Rather than focusing on self-performance, healthcare managers supervise the activities of others. You have a great degree of control over and responsibility for others' activities. Your time is governed by the work activities and needs of your reporting staff, as well as the needs of your organization. Your work is constantly interrupted by people problems, organizational mandates, and change in work direction generated by upper management. Furthermore, your first responsibility is to the individuals you supervise, not to yourself. This means that your priorities and interests often take a backseat.

Autonomy Versus Circumstantial Control

As a healthcare professional, you have autonomous control over your work responsibilities. In many cases, your work activity is primarily governed by a job description, and you perform your tasks based on deadlines, processes, and procedures. Unless an emergency arises, you can work at your own pace and accomplish the goals you desire, based on your own performance and motivation.

As a manager, circumstances and situations control your action flow. The organizational contribution your department makes is the main factor in determining your workflow and your daily responsibilities. As emergencies arise, you must mobilize your entire department and determine who will work to attain specific objectives. Flexibility is a key factor in your success; you must be positively reactive, adaptable, and versatile in undertaking your management responsibilities.

Quantitative Versus Qualitative Outcomes

The roles of most healthcare professionals usually lead to a variety of quantitative outcomes. In general, performance as a professional is assessed based on meeting quantitative outcomes on a regular basis.

For example:

- A laboratory technician conducts analysis and assays, which produces numerical (quantitative) outcomes.
- A staff pharmacist is responsible for filling a set amount of prescriptions on a daily basis.
- A staff nurse has a certain number of procedures and activities that, if successfully undertaken, indicates that you had a good day.

In a similar manner, as a physician you deal largely in quantitative outcomes as well; however, moving to the management billet of a physician leader, measuring your success will be more difficult, as you will begin to work with personalities and perceptions rather than measurable results. Consider that even the most important indicator of successful healthcare management performance—patient satisfaction—is very difficult to measure numerically and is definitely qualitative in scope.

Focusing on Definitive Criteria Versus Focusing on Overall, Comprehensive Goals

Healthcare professionals deal with definite outcomes. For example, you either complete a laboratory analysis or not; fill a prescription correctly, or fail to note contraindications. Having clear-cut criteria provides a degree of satisfaction: You can recognize clearly the contribution you make toward providing stellar health care. Furthermore, this clarity of outcome provides a building block–like sequence, whereby you can improve your performance each day and compare it with a previous goal.

Healthcare management offers few black-and-white performance criteria. Given all the dynamics of change and expectations mentioned earlier in this chapter, it is very difficult to measure performance, clearly identify key performance criteria, and establish reliable goals for optimum performance. As a result, you must adapt your thinking to look at the breadth of activity, as opposed to the depth of activity. This means looking at the big picture as it relates to all of your department's activities, establishing overall, comprehensive goals, and closely monitoring performance with an open mind—all without ever losing sight of the objective of providing excellent health care.

Making Ethical Decisions

Certainly, this dimension of professional responsibility is not a new factor to your work life, as it is the guiding beacon for physician action. Accordingly, the initial decisions required in your role as a physician leader will be made with an already established frame of reference based on your professional experience to date. Numerous guidelines for making ethical decisions exist, but the following 7-step process offers a convenient, concise method for confronting ethical dilemmas.

In particular, the following process serves as a reminder that good decision making typically involves double checking before taking action. For example, the key issue in the checklist may well be Step 6, which requires you (and the organization you're making decisions for) to essentially **look in the mirror** and evaluate the risk of public disclosure of your action and your willingness to bear it.

Step 1: Recognize the ethical dilemma.

Step 2: Get the facts.

Step 3: Identify your options.

Step 4: Test each option: Is it legal? Is it right? Is it beneficial?

Step 5: Decide which option to follow.

Step 6: Double-check your decision by asking two basic questions:

"How would I feel if my family found out about my decision?"

"How would I feel about this if my decision were printed in the local newspaper?"

Step 7: Take action.

UNDERSTANDING COMMON ORGANIZATIONAL STRUCTURES

Formally defined, **organizing** is the process of arranging people and other resources to work together to accomplish a goal. Organizing involves both dividing up the tasks to be performed and coordinating results to achieve a common purpose.

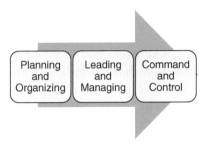

FIGURE 1–2.   The three essentials of action.

Figure 1–2 shows the role that planning and organizing, leading and managing, and command and control play in the management process. As the figure shows, managers are responsible for carrying out plans. Planning activities often precede organizing tasks, but the sequence varies based on the needs and culture of each healthcare organization (Chapter 5 covers the planning process in detail). Many beginning physician leaders will likely first follow long-standing plans and procedures that upper managers or former managers created before creating new plans of their own. Whatever the specifics of your situation, organizing and planning tasks often happen in close conjunction; be flexible and adjust your management duties to suit the situation.

At the most basic level, organizing includes

- Implementing a clear mission, core values, objectives, and strategy
- Identifying who is to do what, who is in charge of whom, and how different people and parts of the organization relate to one another

The challenge of organizing effectively is to choose the best form or structure to fit the demands of a given situation.

The **organization structure** is the system of tasks, workflow, reporting relationships, and communication channels that links the diverse parts of an organization. The specific structures vary greatly between healthcare organizations, but generally, any structure must both allocate or assign tasks and provide for the coordination of performance results.

Unfortunately, talking about good structures is easier than actually creating them. This is why you often read and hear about **restructuring**, the process of changing an organization's structure in an attempt to improve performance.

Organization structures can be described and classified in several ways based on formality, function, divisions, and more.

Formal and Informal Structures

You may know the concept of structure best in the form of an organization chart. A typical **organization chart** identifies, by diagram, key positions and job titles within an organization. It shows the lines of authority and communication between them.

An organizational chart shows the **formal structure**, the intended or official structure. The diagram depicts the way the organization is intended to function. Organizational charts can tell much about an organization, including

- **The division of work:** Positions and titles show how work responsibilities are assigned.
  - **Supervisory relationships:** Lines among positions show who reports to whom.
  - **Communication channels:** Lines among positions show formal communication channels.
  - **Major subunits:** Positions reporting to a common manager are identified as a group.
  - **Levels of management:** Layers of management from top to bottom are shown.

However, behind every formal structure typically lies an **informal structure**. This is a **shadow** organization made up of the unofficial, but often critical, working relationships among organizational members. If you drew an organization's informal structure, it would show who talks to and interacts regularly with whom, regardless of their formal titles and relationships. Informal structures include people meeting for coffee, exercise groups, friendship cliques, and many other possibilities. The lines of informal structures often cut across levels and move from side to side, rather than solely up and down.

Because of the complex nature of organizations and constantly shifting performance demands, informal structures can be very helpful in accomplishing large and small tasks. Through the emergent and spontaneous relationships of informal structures, people gain access to interpersonal networks of emotional support and friendship that satisfy important social needs. They also benefit from contacts with others who can help them better perform their jobs and tasks. Valuable learning and knowledge sharing take place as people interact informally throughout the workday and in a variety of unstructured situations.

Savvy organizations identify and capitalize on their informal structures. For example, a study by the Center for Workforce Development found that the cafeteria can be a "hotbed for informal learning," as workers at a variety of levels tend to share ideas, problems, and solutions with one another over snacks and meals. Dynamic healthcare managers can mobilize these types of informal learning opportunities as resources for organizational improvement.

Of course, informal structures also have potential disadvantages. They can be susceptible to rumor, carry inaccurate information, breed resistance to change, and even divert work efforts from important objectives. People who feel left out of informal groupings may become dissatisfied.

DIVIDING WORK AMONG TEAMS

Formally defined, a team is a small group of people with complementary skills who work together to achieve a shared purpose and who hold themselves mutually accountable for its accomplishment.

Teamwork is the process of people working together to accomplish these goals. The ability to lead through teamwork requires a special understanding of how teams operate and the commitment to use that understanding to help them achieve high levels of task performance and membership satisfaction. One of the biggest benefits of teamwork is **synergy**—the creation of a whole that is greater than the sum of its parts. Synergy occurs when teams use their resources to the fullest and achieve through collective performance far more than is otherwise possible.

An important part of a manager's job is to know when a team is the best organizing choice for a task. The second is to know how to work with and lead the team to best accomplish that task. The following section discusses the first task, using teams as an organizing tool for dividing work responsibilities.

The Benefits of Teams

While synergy is an important advantage, teams are useful in other ways. Being part of a team can have a strong influence on individual attitudes and behaviors. Working in and being part of a team can satisfy important individual needs and also improve performance. Teams, simply put, can be very good for both organizations and their members. Teams can be useful for a variety of reasons, including the following:

- Increasing resources for problem solving
- Fostering creativity and innovation
- Improving the quality of decision making
- Enhancing members' commitments to tasks
- Raising motivation through collective action
- Helping control and discipline members
- Satisfying individual needs as organizations grow in size

Of course, organizing based on a team approach is never a guaranteed success. Who hasn't been part of a team that included members who slacked off because responsibility was diffused among several people and the rest of team would take care of the work? And who hasn't heard people complain about having to attend what they consider to be another **time-wasting** meeting?

Fortunately, things don't have to be this way. In fact, they must not be if teams are to make their best contributions to organizations. The following sections explore some of the most common types of teams in today's workplace and recommends when each type of team is most appropriate.

IDENTIFYING CHARACTERISTICS
OF STRONG TEAMS

As a healthcare manager, establishing a team orientation is important in order to build a progressive work environment.

As a new healthcare manager, you are most likely inheriting a ready-made team. Your department may have been working together under the leadership of your predecessor. Even if you are forming a brand-new team, the following guidelines can help establish the standards you wish to incorporate into your team-building and team-orientation efforts. The following are key qualities consistent in all winning teams:

- A **motivated** team attains its stated mission successfully and effectively. Motivation can come from a variety of sources, the first of which should be the department manager. Motivation can be positive, emphasizing encouragement, and progressive action, or negative, emphasizing less-than-satisfactory consequences due to failure to meet team objectives. Motivation also must come from the work group itself. Individuals must inspire one another to greater performance and support the efforts of all team members. Also, each team member must be self-motivated. Chapter 6 will provide more information on motivation.

- A **credible and respected** team is known for getting the job done. The team earns credibility and commands the respect of patients and other departments. Strong teams have a wide base of technical knowledge and can readily provide whatever level of assistance is needed. Such teams are self-perpetuating, as they attract and retain other strong members.

- A **progressive** team grows continuously and develops expertise in an ongoing effort to enhance quality. Teams become progressive by valuing individual contribution, constantly attaining new technical knowledge, and experimenting with and implementing new methods of practices. Conversely, a **regressive** team loses ground and fails to participate positively in organizational activities, and its members are labeled as losers throughout the organization.

- An **inspired** team is fueled by their will to win. Individual members are success driven, and their leaders reinforce the importance of succeeding. This combination is the basis for inspiration. To keep these teams inspired, clear goals must be established, outcomes must be defined, and methods of attaining success should be delineated by the leader with the participation of all members.

- A **talented and seasoned** team has the skills and abilities needed to achieve a desired end, even if surprises pop up along the way. **Talent** encompasses technical knowledge, performance ability relative to current healthcare mandates, and awareness of business objectives within the context of those mandates.

- An **achievement-oriented** team wants success on an individual, group, and organizational level. In making their contribution, team members must be challenged to become the best they can be. As a manager, you must foster educational development, training opportunities, open communication, and goal attainment for each staff member.

- A **spirited** team is supportive, positive, result-oriented, and winning. These adjectives relate not only to the perceptions others have of the team, but also to something perhaps more important: the team's perception of itself. Losing teams are characterized as discordant, dysfunctional, or negative.

Resilience

Great teams are not defeated by adversity—they bounce back. No team is perfect, but you must remember that no team operates under perfect conditions every day. As a result, adverse situations arise that can have negative and demotivating effects. When these situations occur, call a staff meeting to ask these questions:

- What went wrong?
- How could it have been avoided?
- What have we learned from this?
- What will we do next time given the same circumstances?

By following this sequence, you give everyone an opportunity to learn from their mistakes, avoid reactive (as opposed to proactive) behavior in tough situations, and become more effective in their everyday work activities.

As a healthcare leader, take the lead in this discussion by admitting any mistake you may have made and acknowledging whatever may have caused a problem that was outside your department's power to remedy. This process provides a basis on which to generate progressive discussion, which can help turn negative situations into positive future action.

Encouraging Strong Team Players

Strong healthcare team members possess eight critical characteristics. As a manager or team leader, you should identify these characteristics (and the work-related behaviors associated with them) as well as encourage your team members to further develop.

- **Drive:** Each team member must have a certain amount of drive to attain individual and group goals. He/she does not need to be jump-started every morning or at the beginning of each shift. The drive toward performing strongly, learning and growing every day, being a motivator for others purely by example, expending energy, and applying on-the-job initiative all characterize a stellar team player.

- **Confidence:** All team members should feel self-assured about their technical abilities, as well as their resilience to perform under changing and critical circumstances. A strong player usually radiates confidence about departmental goals and everyday work activities. Patients and fellow workers pick up on this attitude and therefore feel comforted by this individual's presence. They have the conviction that the job will get done and that when the going gets tough—an everyday occurrence in health care—the job will still get done.

- **Discipline:** Good workers are disciplined. They steadily make exact determinations and seek all facts necessary for making the best possible decision. They get the job done correctly the first time and do not cause little problems that can add up to big problems. Good team members know intrinsically what has to be done and how to do it; that is, they set their own objectives and determine a course of action for achieving those objectives with excellence. Their sense of discipline is self-perpetuating throughout the entire department.

- **Desire:** A hunger to get better all the time is a constant motivator for team players. An individual with desire wants to help others and has a strong need to learn and grow on the job. Team members who possess desire do not need to be **hand-fed** with the promise of educational opportunities, promotions, or raises; rather, they seek out learning opportunities every day and are perpetually fueled by this desire to become better at their jobs and stronger in their daily contributions to the organization, team, and patient's health.

- **Dedication:** Strong team members emanate dedication to a common goal for all healthcare workers—to provide stellar health care to all patients. They are equally dedicated to all team goals, departmental objectives, and one another in providing help, guidance, and technical assistance.

- **Acumen:** Every healthcare employee has a certain amount of technical acumen and expertise that they bring to the job. Whether that expertise lies in conducting a good laboratory assay, filling a prescription correctly, or cleaning a patient's room quickly and efficiently, strong team members bring their unique, essential ability to the workplace everyday.

- **Loyalty:** Team loyalty is critical in any workplace, especially in the healthcare industry. Each team member's first loyalty, of course, is to the healthcare institution and its mission of providing care to its patient community. The second loyalty is to the department manager or team leader and is demonstrated by following set objectives, providing feedback, and accomplishing team goals. The third loyalty is to the work group, to act as a positive participant who contributes to group goals. Fourth, the team members maintain a dedication to escalating their individual strong performance and progressive development on the job.

- **Development:** Each team member should desire to grow and develop on the job. This development expands beyond the parameters of basic technical growth: Strong healthcare team members seek to learn more about the healthcare industry and understand the changing dimensions of the business. They know how to interpret the impact of change in the social environment and their communities, and they understand how these changes may affect their particular duties and the institution's mission.

An often-overlooked aspect of team member development is **interpersonal skills**. A strong team member seeks to learn more about others' personalities and professional preferences, relative to job performance. Developing interpersonal skills contributes significantly to an ever-expanding knowledge base from which an employee can grow, prosper, and continuously improve the quantity and quality of their work contribution.

Maintaining and Reinforcing a Strong Team Orientation

Just as establishing a team orientation is not an exact science, keeping a work group committed to and engaged with a team orientation for many months—and perhaps years—is a day-to-day challenge that healthcare managers face.

Numerous strategies are available to help healthcare managers constantly reinforce a team concept within their department. Many hospitals or healthcare organizations have ongoing training programs to help managers continually refine how they motivate their teams and improve efficiency.

The following are some of the most useful strategies:

- **Point team members back to established, common objectives.** All team members need to know the objectives and mission of the department as well as the organization. Remember that management involves asking the right questions. Question your staff about their perceptions as to the main objectives of the department and the common goals toward which individuals should be striving as members of the team.

- **Recognize individual talents and ask for suggestions on how each individual's talent can be applied to the team.** Be a manager who asks team members for individual, unique suggestions and recommendations. The best source for learning how to create synergism between individual talent and group contribution is the individual department member.

- **Maintain two-way feedback.** In addition to providing feedback to your staff on ways they can become better team members, ask team members their opinions on your management style within the team and on the way that the team is progressing toward stated goals.

- **Identify changing dynamics or factors affecting your department as proactively as possible.** While good teams have the ability to handle change, aware managers make the process of responding to change less painful. Again, elicit ideas from your staff about what is changing relative to their jobs and, more importantly, how they can best prepare to handle that change successfully.

- **Be unafraid to reassign.** A team's ability to bounce back from adversity is a hallmark of success. As a healthcare manager, you may have to reassign individuals occasionally to help team members who require extra assistance. Rely on veterans and stronger players to provide assistance. Reassigning not only helps a team achieve objectives, but it can increase team allegiance and individual motivation.

- **Provide opportunities to grow, learn, and develop.** Present as many in-service exercises as possible, and use the expertise within your department to present new ideas to the group. One strategy in this area is to have show-and-tell sessions in which team members explain to each other new principles, strategies, and methods of accomplishing technology-based ends.

- **Establish new goals.** Hold meetings at least once a quarter (or even monthly) to set new goals for the department for continuous improvement. Review past goals and accomplishments, seek explanations for why goals were either achieved or not achieved, and seek input from the group concerning their perceptions as to the achievement of these goals. Make this a group process to ensure credibility as well as maximum input and opportunities for shared knowledge.

Avoiding Groupthink

Among the risks of team decision making is a phenomenon called **groupthink**, the tendency for highly cohesive groups to lose their critical evaluative capabilities. Members of very cohesive teams may publicly agree with actual or suggested courses of action while privately having serious doubts about them. Strong feelings of team loyalty can make it hard for members to criticize and evaluate one another's ideas and suggestions. Desires to hold the team together and avoid disagreements may result in poor decisions. Symptoms that groupthink may be occurring include

- **Having illusions of invulnerability:** Members assume the team is too good for criticism or beyond attack.

- **Rationalizing unpleasant and disconfirming data:** Members refuse to accept contradictory data or consider alternatives thoroughly.

- **Believing in inherent group morality:** Members act as though the group is inherently right and above reproach.

- **Stereotyping competitors as weak, evil, and stupid:** Members refuse to look realistically at other groups.

- **Pressurizing others to conform to group wishes:** Members refuse to tolerate anyone who suggests the team may be wrong.

- **Self-censorship by members:** Members refuse to communicate personal concerns to the whole team.

- **Having illusions of unanimity:** Members accept consensus prematurely, without testing its completeness.

- **Mind guarding:** Members protect the team from hearing challenging ideas or outside viewpoints.

Team leaders and managers can help identify and minimize the effects of groupthink by keeping the following tips in mind:

- Examine and evaluate the entire range of the Spheres of Influence in a force field manner, using the four sectors illustrated in Figure 1–3.

- Assign the role of critical evaluator to each team member; encourage a sharing of viewpoints.

- Do not, as a leader, seem partial to one course of action; do absent yourself from meetings at times to allow free discussion.

- Create subteams to work on the same problems and then share their proposed solutions.

- Have team members discuss issues with outsiders and report back on their reactions.

- Invite outside experts to observe team activities and react to team processes and decisions.

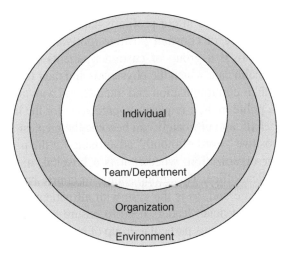

FIGURE 1–3.   The spheres of influence.

THE CUSTOMER/PATIENT PROFILE

An essential element of daily life for both physicians and physician leaders is dealing with the unique customer/patient profile existent in every sector of the American healthcare business arena. As depicted in Figure 1–4, most customer/patients fall into three general behavioral categories, which can also be considered as subcultures. By understanding both the composition groups of the profile and the group norms, the physician leaders can draw on their experience as physicians in dealing with these three-factor sectors, as well as acting as both facilitators and educators to their respective staff in how to most effectively manage healthcare delivery across the span of this profile.

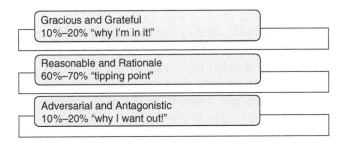

FIGURE 1–4.   The customer/patient profile.

The first group depicted in our profile is naturally the easiest group to deal with and a source of constant positive motivation to all healthcare providers. This cadre is a group of customer/patients who are normally **grateful** for the health care which the physicians and their team provide and are **gracious** in their communication and interactions with all of their care-givers. They are polite in their requests, appreciative for the hard work rendered on their behalf, and ultimately can become the greatest protagonist in promulgating positive "word of mouth" advertising for the position of physicians and their organization, whether it is a hospital, medical staff, or independent medical office. This group should of course be tended to with maximum loving care and, as is the case with all patients, the best health care possible. The physician leaders need to ensure that their staff recognizes the positive role that this particular group of patients plays in the overall business scheme of their operation and make certain that no one in their chain of command takes anyone in this group for granted. The continuity of excellent healthcare service and consistency of clear communication, pride in the office, accountable care provision, and the reinforcement of personal trust between the provider and patient will warranty a sound long-term relationship with this prominent group of customer/patients.

The second group depicted is the segment of customer/patients who can best be described as **reasonable and rational** in their dealings with the physician leaders' organization and again, in their relationship with physicians themselves in their role as primary caregiver. This group is extremely important for three basic reasons. First, this is typically the largest group of customer/patients for any physician-led group; as their basic psychological profile is a willingness to trust the physicians and their staff, these customer/patients follow their counsel, as they believe that the physician and the other care providers are the **experts** in the healing process, and while being wary, they are at least initially trusting in the dealings with their care providers. By definition, this would suggest that they would indeed be the largest group of customer/patients. Second, this group can be the **tipping point** group, as suggested by thought leaders such as Malcolm Gladwell, as they are the middle swing group in this profile and can gravitate toward the bottom group (not good, as we will see in the coming paragraphs) or elevate to the top group and become among the physician-led group's most prominent supporters. Third, this group based on its size and diversity is the most complex group and would exhibit the widest range of behavior, mandating that the physicians encourage each and every one of their staff members to understand that a **one size fits all** approach to dealing with customer/patients would be particularly perilous with this group.

Accordingly, the physician leader should activate five strategies aimed at the particular nuances of this group but keep good principles for dealing with all customer/patients. These five strategies can be considered house rules and are equally applicable to a medical office setting as they are to any physician-led business environment such as a hospital setting or similar venue of health care. They are as follows:

1. Listen ardently, actively, and effectively to each patient; seek to know the essential answers to what they need immediately.

2. Learn as much as possible from the patient at the outset of their arrival in our office and strive to garner two or three major action points leading to effective and efficient treatment.

3. Lead the patient to the area of our office or facility where they can most quickly and positively get the treatment that they need.

4. Laugh in concert with the patient at any opportunity to ensure comfort, compassion, and empathy; do not laugh or joke with the patient if it is possible that it might be misconstrued as sarcasm.

5. Link the patients to help them as quickly as possible, and establish a link to get help and assistance to the patient at any time as needed, getting the patient all that they require.

While appearing elemental in a book and certainly with the employ of alliteration by using the letter *L*, these five house rules can assist in the caregiving process for this significant middle group which in the final analysis could be the most important group of customer/patients.

The final group depicted in our diagram consists of patients who often fall into the roles of being antagonists and adversaries to the physicians and their staff members. This group might only consist of 10% to 20% of the overall composition of customer/patients, but unfortunately due to their behavior, this might in fact be the most time consuming and certainly difficult to manage in a healthcare setting. Like the nonplayers discussed in the management section of this text, it is unlikely that the behavior of this particular group will ever change; unfortunately, their needs for good health care will not diminish and from a crass business perspective, they are paying customers. There are four essential strategies that the physician leaders should use as a primary caregiver and as teaching points to their staff:

1. **Do not argue with antagonistic/adversarial customer/patients.** Show them the facts, use records as needed, and always get an assist.

2. **Focus on the objective and unemotional.** Try to stay cool, calm, and collected when dealing with these individuals, and always use a medical record or other written documents to be the focus of discussions, rather than engaging in conjecture or subjective viewpoints (no matter how tempting).

3. **Work backstage as much as possible.** Many medical office practice managers suggest that customer/patients of this ilk **love to put on a show.** Accordingly, use any opportunity available to have discussions with these individuals not in the main office lobby or reception area, but in a private office or other space away from the potential **audience** of other customer/patients, several of which might be concordant adversaries/advocates among your patient group.

4. **Get assistance at any time.** While it is time consuming for doctors to stop what they are doing or upset their schedules to deal with these types of individuals, they can often be a wise investment of time to nip problems instigated by these individuals as quickly as possible. Often, the physician is listening to the initial lament of the agitator/antagonist and then pledging more specific discussion of treatment at the earliest convenience of the physician is all that is needed, as it disposes of the perpetual lament of the antagonist/agitator that **no one is listening to me.**

These strategies should be used not only with the agitator/antagonist, but also with any patients in our middle group who exhibit overly emotional behavior. In fact, all the strategies in this section are not exclusive to one group and can be used from a situational perspective based on individual behavior rather than categorical assumption.

ESSENTIAL TENETS OF LEADERSHIP

The essential tenets for successful leaders are founded on basic principles which in general can be applied to any profession or work role, but have particular relevance to a physician or healthcare leader. As depicted in Figure 1–5, the imperative elements are ability, motivation, and knowledge. Working in concert, they can become the foundations for success in any profession; however, a lack of substance in any one of these areas can lead to abject failure in any profession and most notably of that of a physician leader.

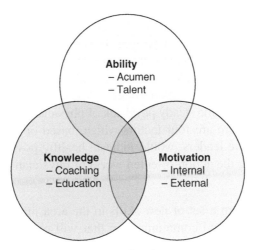

FIGURE 1–5.   Critical components of performance.

The first factor is ability, which for our purposes is defined as a capability of achieving performance through basic skills, intrinsic talent, and appropriate application of the work personality characteristics which we will delineate in our chapter about leadership. Simply put, ability addresses the **can do** potential of the new physician leader to assume the roles of leader, facilitator, visionary, educator, and manager. This can be based on previous experience in both health care and informative experiences in school and can be depicted as the apparent ability that the new physician leader brings to the equation on **Day 1**. The questions of "Can this new leader motivate their staff?," "Does this new leader have the skills to communicate new ideas, set goals, and important objectives to all constituents and staff?," and "Is this new leader capable of understanding and managing the budgets, people, and care equation of their new assignment?" need to be posed pro-actively and progressively. The answers to these essential questions can be an accurate reflection of the new physician leader's preeminent ability in their new role.

The second factor in our matrix of essential tenets of physician leadership is motivation, which can be simply defined as the aspirant leader's desire to **want to** do the job. Motivation, of course, can be based on many factors: money, ego, self-esteem, and an array of other factors which can be seen from a positive perspective starting with the pioneering thoughts on motivation of Abraham Maslow and his hierarchy of needs. Equally, motivation can be based on a set of negative factors which can apply even to physician leadership. For example, a physician might be burnt out on the rigors of being an emergency room physician and decides that physician leadership might offer a greener pasture. Relatedly, the constantly diminishing reimbursement scheme (and that's probably the right word for it) of Medicaid and Medicare could easily give a physician something to run from, namely a diminishing bank account that is in a constant state of fluctuation, and run toward the steady paycheck of physician leadership.

Accordingly, there are four factors which, based on success profiles of current healthcare leaders, would indicate healthy positive motivating factors for entering the action-oriented world of physician and healthcare leadership:

1. A desire to learn a set of new skills in the area management, strategy, leadership, and communication that will positively impact the overall delivery of health care within a particular community

2. A strong commitment to expanding the abilities of the physicians in the interest of developing all of their individual strengths—spiritual, mental, and physical—in a pursuit of excellence in the interest of helping nurses, staff members, and other healthcare professionals from a leadership perspective

3. An intrinsic desire to be the person who makes the big decisions, leads the action, maintains accountability for outcomes and results, innovates the vision for the overall direction of health care within their assigned sector, and ultimately is the person who is in charge of the most precious product in a free society, health care, and medicine

4. An unwavering interest in human behavior, as a major distinction between being a physician dealing with one patient at a time and a physician leader dealing with a multitude of people in multiple personalities (sometimes in the same individual) is based overwhelmingly in human behavior and basic psychology

These four motivation points can act as a functional checklist for anyone considering physician or healthcare leadership as a career direction, and post-decision, as a criteria list for the individual physician leader's sense of job satisfaction, which in itself is a major motivational factor.

The third factor in our essential tenets of physician leadership is that of knowledge, which we will define as the physician leaders' **know how** relative to the job. Knowledge can take many shapes and semblances; a variety of knowledge is required for success as a physician leader. Business knowledge is important, as a healthcare leader must know how to make budgets, formulate strategic plans, and often contribute to the marketing and promotion of a medical or healthcare organization. Emotional intelligence is extremely important, as a physician who is clinically strong but lacks basic apathy and is consistently incapable of understanding the views, perspectives, and emotionalism of those around him/her should stay a clinician and not become a physician leader. Emotional intelligence is in fact simply **people smarts** and being a leader requires that you know your people well so that you can motivate them toward their highest level of efficacious performance. This aspect of knowledge might be the most important tenet to not only be present on the first day, but constantly honed by continuous education and acquisition of new methods of leading or managing people.

Organizational knowledge is also important, as the physician leader must know the strengths, weaknesses, opportunities, and threats (SWOT) of their organization so that they can address the strengths, the weaknesses, take positive and aggressive advantages of the opportunities at hand, and minimize, if not totally negate, the threats to the organization.

All three tenets—ability, motivation, and knowledge—should be inventoried by the physician leader and perhaps by a trusted mentor as a decision to enter physician leadership is considered. Furthermore, once in the role of a leader, all of these tenets should be constantly, purposefully, and consistently reinforced and upgraded in the interest of achieving maximum effectiveness.

THE MISTAKE REVIEW MATRIX

A major responsibility for a physician leader is to take responsibility appropriately and set corrective action when a mistake is made. Ineffective leaders in any capacity too often take deleterious action which can actually exacerbate the negative impact of a mistake made by leaders or their charges. For example, the leader can deny that the mistake was never made, which can quickly negate trust with their staff. From another perspective, the leader can engage in the **blame game** and lay the fault and genesis for the mistake at the feet of another department, circumstance, top leadership of the organization, or any other of a number of potential antagonists. The leaders can lose trust when they minimize the mistake and its impact, or from a converse perspective, blow it out of proportion—in one case, making a mountain out of a molehill, and in the other, a molehill into a mountain. In both cases, the perspective on the action which causes the mistake is distorted and the likelihood of a corrective action in the future is minimized. Naturally, other maladies can exist when healthcare leaders do not handle mistakes made by their team collectively, or by the leader individually, in a constructive and appropriate manner by repeating the mistakes, not learning from the mistakes, or letting the mistake become fodder for negative gossip which sow the seeds of group mistrust for the leader.

Four steps should be taken by a physician leader when a mistake is made in the interest of amending the negative impact and for setting a more progressive and positive course for future action, as demonstrated in Figure 1–6. To begin with, the leader should set a specific time to discuss the mistake with either a set of individuals who were responsible for the mistake or those who took part in action which led to the miscue. This can be an individual or a small meeting, or if appropriate, include every member of a particular department or organization. Whenever possible, individuals who did not have anything to do with the mistake, especially those who would seize on the opportunity to ignorantly embellish the negativity of the mistake without first-hand knowledge of what actually happened should be excluded from a mistake review meeting.

With the right group assembled, the physician leader should start out with a review of what happened to cause the mistake, with the augmentation that this is strictly the leader's perspective. Using a tight composition of three to five essential points to illustrate what happened as factually and efficiently as possible, the leader presents a step-by-step progression that reviews the action leading to a mistake. In doing so, he/she will likely be able to bring focus to the particular step which caused the entire miscue. During this process, the leader should look to his/her superstars and action agents among his/her group to provide

1. Here's **what happened,** in as much as I can tell from my vantage point.	2. Here's **why it happened,** as simply as I can tell, cold and true.
3. Next time, **we will do** _____, and **I will do**_____.	4. From this, I **learned**_____, and **we learned** _____.

FIGURE 1–6.   Mistake Review Matrix.

supporting detail as well, as they are constructive individual perspective on what occurred.

Second, the leader should then turn their attention to why they thought the problem happened and why the mistake occurred. The leader should give a brief analysis of the problem, a particular inefficiency that took place, or as is all too common, a human error factor intrinsic to the mistake at hand. This analysis should be specific and to the point and should not needlessly wander theoretically or become too **touchy-feely** in nature. Again, the incorporation of comments, observations, and suggestions from members of the staff who are positive advocates and clearly proven superstars in the group makes this segment of the mistake review—and indeed, the whole process—resonant, responsible, and realistic.

Third, the leaders should state unequivocally what he will do in the next time a similar situation or assignment akin to the one centric to the mistake being discussed occurs. Of course, this will bring a new set of actions which will support the basic premise of Einstein's supposition that the definition of insanity is doing the same thing twice and expecting a different result. Rather, as attested to by Frederick Winslow Taylor, it will present a new system for the future, for his adage astutely reminds the leader, **"the system which you have in place today is perfectly suited only for the results that you're getting today."**

The declaration of an improved strategy to contend with the challenge of the circumstances exempted by the mistake at hand is not only to clearly communicate to the leaders a resolution to a **better way**, but additionally reinforce the trust of the majority of their staff that they are accountable and enlightened in what is going on as well as what we are going to do to perform a better job in the future. This phase of this process should also include the leader's ideas for correcting group action for moving forward and confronting similar circumstances. This is a wonderful opportunity for the leader again to engage the participation of the additives and superstars, and his/her group is a progressive and improved solution specific to the situation at hand and from a more general perspective, a demonstrated encouragement of true participatory management with the solid citizens among his/her group of charges.

Finally, the mistake review matrix provides a terrific opportunity for the physician leader to enact a learning organization semblance to retain. By stating what he/she believes the team has learned from the experience, as well as—and perhaps even leading with—what he/she has learned from the experience, an opening emerges to do some real on-the-job learning. In acting as a lead educator, the healthcare leader in this case can garner a set of learning points specific not only to his/her charge as physician leader, but hopefully a set of learning points that will be commenting constructive to the entire group. In doing so, the physician leader to ensure that every day becomes an opportunity to learn something new to the benefit of the entire group, and every mistake is an opportunity to learn a better strategy, and that mistakes are not repeated while the knowledge reaped from their occurrence is harvested to move the entire group forward.

THE CRITICAL THREE DEPARTURE QUESTIONS

One of the more important responsibilities of the leader in any regard is appropriate self-management to ensure that stress does not become pejorative or counterproductive in your daily accountabilities. Accordingly, it should come as no shock that self-created stress can become a major malady for a physician leader, particularly in the initial segment of their responsibilities as a new leader. As truly **driven** individuals—some would say, "Type A personalities"—physicians in general could become victims of self-created stress, and when combining the additional responsibilities of leadership and management, the paradox of not taking care of oneself relative to stress can occur while pursuing the quest of taking care of your new staff and work team.

The use of three departure questions—labeled as such because you will ask them yourself as you depart the workplace and head home—can help negate unnecessary self-created stress (Figure 1–7).

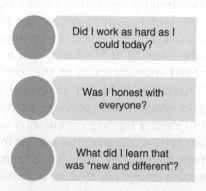

Did I work as hard as I could today?

Was I honest with everyone?

What did I learn that was "new and different"?

FIGURE 1–7.   Charting daily progress.

Question 1   Did I work as hard as I could today?

This question helps the new physician leader ascertain if they put forth maximum effort throughout the entire day. This is something which is eminently within your own control and also is a leading indicator to your staff and constituents about your level of dedication.

Question 2   Was I honest with everyone?

As we have discussed, trust is an absolutely imperative factor between a leader and his/her team. If trust is abridged or even perceived as being compromised, it will be difficult if not impossible for it to be regained at maximum level. Being honest with everyone has become in the leadership argot the factor of **transparency** not only in organizations but also within the political sphere and thus likely part of the consciousness of your staff members. So at the end of each day, it is useful to do a quick self-examination about how candid you were in all of the communication to your staff, peers, and superiors.

Being honest with everyone also encompasses delivering bad news as quickly and as appropriately direct as possible. Using the expression, **cold and true** can help in delivering bad news. For example, if you are charged with telling your staff that a significant amount of paperwork must be regenerated to get ready for a joint commission inspection, an effective communication strategy would be to say, "Folks, I have to tell you, cold and true, that we must redo all the paperwork we thought was all set for the upcoming inspection. I know it's a grind, but we have a firm grip now on what is needed so at least we will only have to do it one more time. So let's get mad, let's get over it, and let's get this done so we could move on to focusing our efforts on what we need to do and what we like to do which is taking care of our patients."

This approach reduces the dramatics, is direct in approach, and allows for immediate emotionalism which can be replaced quickly with necessary, reasoned action.

Question 3   What did I learn today that was new and different?

The opportunity to learn something new is available every day within a healthcare workplace. Patients can provide new information such as widely held perceptions about health care or a particular concern among the community which can be valuable when constructing strategy of providing care. Staff members can offer input based on the depth of knowledge that they possess about their particular area of the operation which

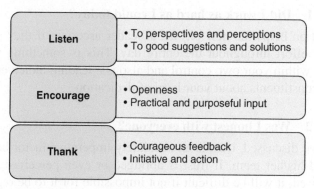

FIGURE 1–8.   **LET** it come to you.

can be useful in making operational plans and perhaps providing quality upgrades relative to the continuing care. And of course, there are the traditional avenues of new information and knowledge from conferences, reliable sources on the Internet, professional journals, and other sources of data and information which can be incorporated into the daily conduct of your medical operation. Therefore, every day represents an opportunity to learn something which will give you an edge both as a leader as well as provide an advantage to your assigned area of responsibility. The attainment of new knowledge every day—at least one new fact, figure, insight, idea, or solution—should not only be part of your takeaway package each day, but be an objective pursued on a daily basis in the interest of personal development and organizational growth. Resisting the **Type A** tendency to try to provoke quick answers and immediate action, it might be useful to **let** some communication come to you, as demonstrated in Figure 1–8 and the **LET Formula**.

The bad news about this triad of questions is that they represent probably the only areas that you control completely—your dedication and work ethic, your honesty and integrity, and your thirst for new knowledge. The good news is if progress is achieved every day in all three of these areas, your leadership will become resilient, your communication will be resonant, and you will enjoy the benefits of professional and personal growth. In the long run, that will not only counteract negative stress, but also bolster the positive action and progressive development of your leadership capacity and management capabilities.

CHAPTER TWO

The PACT System for Strategic Leadership Communication

*W*e too often forget that the truth in all matters, is that in the end all that matters is that Good is the greatest force of all.

- W. Somerset Maugham

INTRODUCTION

All healthcare leaders rely on communication as the essential tool in setting plans, getting results, and continuously developing their staff. In our work with healthcare leaders, we have learned many lessons which are not only effective in the unique healthcare business arena, but have been translated across to professions such as school administration and corporate organizations. In this chapter, we will explore a practical strategy for maximizing strategic leadership communication copyrighted as the PACT System. This system has not only been validated through field use over the past 20 years in an array of organizations, but more importantly, it is an intuitive system which can be readily understood and practically applied immediately to your organization and specific leadership responsibilities.

The PACT acronym stands for the four essential values that are expected in all leadership communication, and indeed, as centric elements of organizational strategy—pride, accountability, commitment, and trust. Each value is augmented by a set of couplets that portray the **pros and cons** of specific action relative to the value, in essence, what happens when a leader adheres to the constructive, positive aspect of a particular factor, and the liabilities and fallacy of inadvertently employing the negative, regressive side of the particular tenet. The chapter is premised on a handbook of over 500 PACT Factors currently employed by the physician leadership cadre of New Jersey's largest medical and healthcare systems, as well as many sectors of the Veterans Administration Health System. We have selected for you the most prominent and universal strategies in the hope that a number of them will have immediate value in your specific situation, as is the intent of this entire book. As you will soon see, they are logical in construct, easy to grasp, and very practical in their application regardless of your particular leadership role, as they are all based on the real world of strategic leadership communication that we work in every day.

THE PERFORMANCE MATRIX

In order to put this chapter in context, we begin with the performance matrix (see Figure 2–1), which depicts the basic three performance categories of any work team. **Superstars**, or action agents, drive the action and are the exemplars of a work unit. They thrive on change, lead the action, define excellence within the organization, act as positive charismatic physician leaders, and fully support the team's goals and organization's mission through their performance. They need little encouragement, but should not be taken for granted. Accordingly, the physician leader should apply the first component of each PACT Factor to the superstar and provide sound direction, full support, maximum available resources, and sound communication to the superstar.

The next group illustrated in the diagram is the **silent majority** of **steady or organizational advocates**. This is the most important group to a physician leader and should be the main focus of organizational communication, as they represent the largest cadre of the team and organization and represent the most dynamic constituency of the healthcare leader, as they are the most able to change and fluctuate in performance based on situation and circumstance. One of the basic maxims of the performance matrix is to manage and lead the steadies in the same way as the superstars—that is,

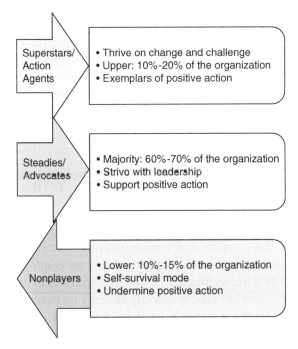

FIGURE 2–1.   The performance matrix.

treat the steadies like superstars and over time, they will start performing and exhibiting the same stellar work behavior as the superstars. With that in mind, the strategic leader should incorporate the first (or primary) component of each PACT Factor in their daily communication, and avoid the nefarious effect of the second (or counter) component.

The third and final populace of the performance matrix is the nonplayer, or organizational agitator and instigator. This group, thankfully, is the smallest in terms of size, but unfortunately can take the majority of the physician leader's communication effort and basic management time. Trying to get the nonplayer, who is self-motivated and self-absorbed to change and become an organizational advocate, can be a thankless and often fruitless endeavor. To minimize that waste of precious time and effort—which can be more productive and efficacious when directed to the superstars and steadies—the physician leader should avoid falling into the traps evident in the second counter component of each PACT Factor. By adhering to the primary component, the strategic physician leader ensures that the superstars and steadies get the support, motivation, and direction through well-calibrated communication that they need, and the nonplayers in turn clearly understand the expectations of the organization not only relative to the **what** is expected in terms of performance and work behavior, but moreover, understand cogently the **how** of the organization—that is, the expectation for daily interpersonal conduct and the standards for pursuing excellence in the interest of providing maximum service to the organization's constituency.

APPLYING THE PACT FACTORS

With the performance matrix in mind, the PACT Factors, which set a foundation for the creation and reinforcement of pride, accountability, commitment, and trust, are viable starting points for employing the PACT System. These four major themes can be applied directly in your workplace and underscored in your leadership strategy by examining the dipolar tendencies (first the right tendency in leadership style and strategy, the second listing the converse/negative tendency) for each of the four major PACT elements. The PACT Formula has a basic philosophy (Figure 2–2) that when encouraged by the physician leader can inspire increased performance and confident, progressive individual staff member action.

Building Pride

Moving from the general applications of the PACT Formula apparent in the preceding paragraphs to specific applications under its acronymic aegis, we will now put more PACT Factors into practice, starting with

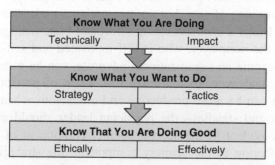

FIGURE 2–2.   PACT knowledge and philosophy.

factors and strategies specific to the building of pride in an organization through strategic leadership communication. Pride is best defined for our purposes as a sentiment shared by the overall majority of the organization or team that

-We are here to perform a vital service.

-We believe that we do our jobs individually and collectively as well as anyone in our field.

-We will always do whatever it takes to take good care of our customers.

-We are in the game to win, not just to play.

This Is Now Versus That Was Then

With the continuing need to change within an organization, based on ever-escalating customer expectations, ever-emergent new technology, and ever-intensifying pace of action, it is easy for the nonplayers to lament current pressures and long for the **good old days**. As is always the case, they can often enlist the more pliable members of the steady group, and create a sense of doubt about current initiatives and organizational direction. It therefore becomes an intrinsic responsibility of the physician and healthcare leader to constantly educate his/her team about current objectives and future goals, all supplemented with a focus on current demands. **Then** or the **good old days** has relatively nothing to do with present-day demands, yet can be a wistful seditious inspiration for the nonplayers and their sympathetic listeners.

To do this, communication in department meetings should include at least one mention of a current event that is directly impacting the organization's current work. An example of this would be the latest government initiative to provide Medicaid and Medicare reimbursement based on patient satisfaction scores. A physician leader who uses an article from a local paper on this current miasma—and that would be readily available, given its prominence—can then link it to the requisites of a medical office to ensure that every action taken **onstage** in view of patients is **customer friendly** and provides the best effort to provide clear communication and compassionate care right from the patient's entry into the front office.

This Is Us Versus That Was Them

Closely related to the preceding facet, healthcare leaders must constantly affirm that they are satisfied with the construct of their current team and fully confident in their abilities. This is essential as the nonplayer will reference the past, in which budgets allowed larger staffs and, undoubtedly, more human resources in general that are available now in the era of **doing more with less to the point of doing everything with nothing**. Citing the wins and notable accomplishments of the current staff, both in a group context and with specific individual, positive recognition is an easy tool that is always available—but often not fully utilized—by physician leaders in their daily communication.

Meaningful Versus Miasma

A good technique to ensure attention in organizational communication is to use a word that is not often heard in management parlance. This gets the staff's attention and can become a nice game among the superstars and steadies, as if the selection is interesting, which can in turn be used as a reference point in ongoing discussion. An example of this is the word, **miasma**, which generally can be defined as a deliberate, self-perpetuating foggy environment. Nonplayers love to create miasma through rumor, innuendo, and sheer mendacity. Focus on the current objectives of the team is the first step; however, the physician leader must strive to always frame the **why** of what the team means to achieve every day and at every opportunity. A simple cause-effect semblance is the best method for this.

For example, the practice of walking a new patient to not only the department that will provide primary service, but additionally introducing them to the first person in the continuum of care resonates maximum meaning to the patient entry process. It also eliminates the always-present potential of a new patient becoming confused and losing trust immediately by getting lost in a facility as they try to independently negotiate the miasma of paperwork and the often-vexing physical layout of a medical facility.

Focus Versus Fissure

As depicted in Figure 2–3, superstars are selfless in nature and understand that by taking care of the customer/patient, their teammates, and the organization's objectives, they are in essence taking good care of themselves. The diagram provides an overview of the triad of their success strategy, which makes them natural leaders in conducting the action needed by the organization and directed by their physician leaders. Nonplayers, on the other hand, are self-centered and seek to create cracks in

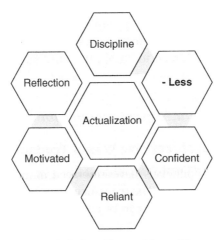

FIGURE 2–3. The positive **self-**.

the overall structure—fissure—and particularly in the semblance of their assigned work team.

The physician leader must therefore keep a focus on team objectives and goals and not allow inappropriate and disproportionate time to be spent on discussing individual problems and issues presented—and all too often, conceived in fiction in a fractious manner—by the nonplayer. Two specific strategies are needed herein. First, the physician leader should take the time in group meetings to provide the **facts** in the face of any prominent rumor in the interest of curbing further conflation by the nonplayer. This should be done crisply and resolutely, and be centered on the true facts, even if that means conveying that a decision has not been made (which is better, for example, than a rumor that a decision has been made that will negatively impact the work group) or simply confirming some bad news as fact. In the latter case, the physician leaders should provide action plans so that their group has an objective to work toward to deal with the **bad news**; that is, the physician leaders should give their group something to run toward, rather than **run from** various negative aspects, both real and perceived.

A second strategy is to implement a house rule that all staff members should provide solutions to all problems encountered by team. The staff should be tasked to innovate solutions, with the leader's guidance, that not only assuages the problem at hand but implements action which is proactive, progressive, pertinent to the situation at hand, and provides a definite, positive payoff for the customer, organization, and team. Naturally, the superstars and steadies of the group will be able to contribute, if not lead, this discussion and maintain a focus on shared direction and action. The nonplayer will be forced to enjoin that discourse positively, or in a very real sense, deal themselves out of the action.

Encouraging Accountability

Transformative Versus Trudging

It is unfortunate that politicians have embraced as part of their pedantic polemic the notion that they will be **transformative leaders** once they attain office, and all too often, become part of a trudging, status quo of inefficacy and mistrust. However, if taken from a more effective venue, a leader who uses a strategy, both in their communication and planning, that is transformative can garner the full support of all of their superstars and the overwhelming majority of their steadies. Transformative leaders are ones who can enact significant change that benefits the organization, customer community, specific work teams, and individual staff members. They can position all of these constituencies in a clearly improved position for the future while leading short-term change catalytically and with maximum outcomes.

As is the case with any sound leadership strategy, the foundation of planning at the team level should start with the staff members who are **closest to the action** and thus are a boundless front for new ideas that could translate into winning practical and pragmatic strategy.

The physician leaders who ask for the **idea of the week** at regular meetings and utilize a daily strategy of asking staff members a simple but very efficient question—"What do you think about (a given objective, new plan, or apparent need for action)?"—are those who are certain to have a ready lode of useful information in formulating new plans of action that will be transformative for their organization. Additionally, a natural level of commitment is at hand, as the genesis of the plan came from the staff that must now support the plan with action. Pride is engendered as results abound from the new action, each individual is assigned an accountability for specific action to support the group objective and results are realized from a smarter, better way of doing things—which, in reality, is a very credible application and definition of transformative action.

Victors Versus Victims

Superstars and steadies want their team to win. As simple as this seems, one only has to consider their devotion to selfless service, which in turn

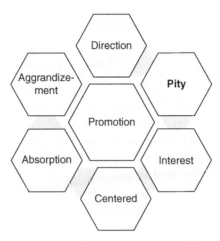

FIGURE 2–4.   The nonplayer **self-**.

will ultimately provide a sense of satisfaction and achievement on their job. The nonplayer conversely wallows in multitudinous excuses and limitless reasons for why the organization and the team are not prepared, ready nor able to take care of business at a top level. The nonplayers unfortunately can take umbrage in the mass media depictions of the **culture of complaint** that exists in American society at large and has been aptly captured in several books and apparent on any talk show (Figure 2–4).

Being a victim is almost trendy, and most nonplayers have that role down to an art form. Unfortunately, their whining and inappropriate emotionalism can be a morale buster, and it must be arrested by the strategic healthcare leader forthrightly and resolutely.

Two strategies can accomplish this. First, the healthcare leader should think of teams that they have been part of which have been successful, as well as notable teams from the world of sports and other organizations that can be used as positive exemplars. This can be done most optimally as a group exercise with the team, as it would then be notable, resonant, and **jointly owned** when ratified and put into action. Three to five aspects of the winning team's composition should be aligned toward specific group's charter. An example of this approach would be to use the sports example of the **underdog** 2012 Super Bowl Champion New York Football Giants as a model, who succeeded through the employs of four criteria:

-Unconditional belief in their abilities rather than what the **expert media** believed

-Planning their work, and then working their plan

-Adjusting their plan as needed, but all while keeping the main objective in mind

-Knowing that the pressure would be on, but not getting on each other when the pressure was on

Taking a closer look at these factors, it is easy to see how an emergency room team in a community hospital, for example, could easily apply these tenets to their daily work. In doing so, the superstars and steadies would have a clear plan to victory (read: positive outcomes) and the nonplayers would be self-exempting if they decided to complain without merit, or bring up problems without solutions while the rest of the department dedicated itself to building an emergency services department that they could truly be proud of every day at work.

Resonance Versus Dissonance

Pride can be built on having a credo—that is, a set of beliefs—that the entire work group can embrace and employ through action. This credo must resonate—echo positively—through the entire work group. The fracturing of communication known as dissonance can be destructive in any work situation, and in some healthcare situations, can actually be dangerous if it leads to miscued action, inaction, or mistakes in treatment. The nonplayer can often create dissonance that can lead to miscommunication deliberately just to **get attention** in a despicable manner; regardless of the motivation, dissonance over time can lead to a schism within a work group, which ultimately can lead to abject failure.

A basic credo should therefore be forwarded by the physician leader, ideally with easy-to-remember phrases, to have a resonant communication of the basic mission and philosophy of the work group. The use of alliteration, repetition of phrasing, and other communication devices helps to facilitate reference and recall of the credo. The following is an example of a credo that the author helped create for a Veterans Administration Medical Clinic in Appalachia:

-The Veteran Patient has served our nation with high distinction, now we have an opportunity to respond in kind.

-The Veteran Patient drives our clinic, not vice versa.

-The Veteran Patient is a neighbor of ours and from a family like mine, so only the best possible care will do.

-The Veteran Patient can do without a lot of noise, hassle, paper chase, or waiting.

-The Veteran Patient will appreciate all that we can do and will be eternally grateful if we can get it all done.

The use of argot familiar to the team, as well as the service community, is essential to making certain that the credo resonates at full force. Furthermore, a well-conceived credo can have long-term usage for a team and act as a long-term warranty of pride in the workplace for the superstars, steadies, and for the person at the top of the organizational chart—the customer.

Garnering Maximum Commitment

Understood/Respected Versus Liked/Accepted

This particular factor is one that finds its fulcrum in the physician leaders themselves as opposed to being a group calculus. Starting with the counter component with any leader wanting to be **liked and accepted,** it is easy to see the fallacy of action relative to nonplayers, whose favorite response to a negative performance evaluation is to say to their physician leaders, **you're doing this to me because you don't like me!** While all of us would want to be liked in general and accepted by those we encounter in a given day, physician leaders charged with the responsibility of moving others toward good work cannot aspire to being socially popular or perceived as being a good egg as a primary goal. The bad news is that the nonplayers, who are usually socially manipulative if nothing else, will use the physician leaders' penchant for being liked as a munificent opportunity to ply that brand of manipulation. The good news in this case is that the superstars and steadies will like the physician leader on an interpersonal basis if the leader seeks to be understood and respected in their job.

There are four steps that a physician leader should take to make certain that respect and understanding take precedence over being liked and accepted.

1. **Get bad medicine done quickly.** New physician leaders should make all of the necessary but somewhat painful actions that are needed in a new department to be done quickly and within the first 3 months on a job. This signals clearly to their staff that they have the fortitude to get the job done and will make tough call as needed.

2. **Bad news doesn't get better with age.** Sitting on bad news doesn't make it go away, nor make it less deleterious, nor give fate and fortune an opportunity to magically revert its circumstances. Using the preface, "I have to tell you something, cold and true," and then delivering the message conveys to a staff member or group that we will get upset about the bad news, get over it, devise a plan of action together and then as a team, get on with it.

3. **Keep the small talk small.** In the New York Metropolitan area, believe it or not, office places can become communicatively hostile during any occasion in which the Yankees find themselves playing their crosstown neighbors, the Mets. Television shows baseball, the stock market, and politics are all avocations and areas of interest which in proper context can be stress relievers on the job, ideally on coffee breaks and at lunch time. The leader who overindulges in conversation on these topics can be seen in the wrong light and cause unneeded discordance and adversity. For example, a Mets fan in a group of Yankee fans, or a conservative working with a bevy of MSNBC viewers could make personal preferences a source of discord if those affiliations became more of a topic of conversation than the work mission at hand.

4. **Manage off-time wisely.** A new manager at a hospital decided to use Facebook as a communication forum for a number of social activities—and unfortunately became **friends** with many of his/her staff. The nonplayers, as you probably already surmised, used this as a prime opening to bring personal lives into the workplace inappropriately. A wealth of precious communication and work time was then dedicated to resolving and remedying some of the prattle from that banal, numbskull source of social media than an upcoming commission inspection of his/her healthcare team's facility. Short answer—stay off of social media, as well as oversocializing with staff members. The superstars and steadies aren't really interested—the nonplayers are interested only to the extent that they can use it against their (in this case, soon to be erstwhile) physician leader.

Gospel Versus Gossip

A pernicious undercurrent can exist in any work group in which gossip takes precedence over more substantial communication. Nonplayers can often be sardonically artful purveyors of gossip, and as lead gossip mongers, they can find any number of steadies willing to give their babble a hearing. Unfortunately, human nature is predisposed to the prurient and as we all know, **bad news sells** in all forms of the media. Taken together, gossip can find a disproportionate place in the workplace, as people want to know the **latest dish** regardless of its relative validity or the veracity of its communicator. This is especially true when a workplace has experienced a tremendous amount of change or a significant downturn in business; in health care, for example, gossip around the facility can feature pending layoffs, closing of units, and an assortment of many other doom and gloom scenarios. The worst impact of this type of communication is the manner in which it promulgates fear among staff and customers; in the former, the steadies can be prime victims of this gossip/ fear mongering, and with the latter, a direct loss of business can occur as people wonder, "Will this organization stay in business?," or perhaps worse, "How does this place stay in business?," as that sentiment goes directly to an at least perceived lack of integrity within the organization. Taken as a net effect, it is difficult to be proud of an organization that rivals the worst in reality television relative to contrived subplots and character exploitation.

To combat this undertow that can undercut the essence of their team, the physician leaders can incorporate the smart address and disposal of rumors at their staff meetings at least once a month. In this as a special item, **The Rumor of the Month**, the physician leader should select a topic which has been apparent gossip fodder, and discuss whether the rumor is true or more likely, why it is not true. By taking the lead in acknowledging that the rumor exists and then minimizing its impact by presenting an action plan, if there is an element of truth, the steadies are provided with a clear choice on who to believe between their physician leaders and the gossipmongers. Additionally, it demonstrates to all of the staff that the physician leader is **clued in** to what the concerns of the staff might be and is willing to **take on** the nonplayer, who is usually also a verbal bully in addition to being a mendacious, disingenuous communicator. The physician leader should crisply address the rumor, confirm its relative truth or counter it with the facts, and then move on to the next topic at hand in the meeting. He/she should not address additional questions specific to the rumor, nor address additional rumors if asked by the nonplayer, but instead say, "I think that most of us agree that we have too much work to do around here without wasting time on every single rumor that is concocted by a few people."

Trust—Encouraging the Individual as the Nucleus of Action

Cascade of Commitment Versus Niagara of Negativity

The nonplayer loves to dwell in negativity; it has been often noted that most nonplayers would not be happy in heaven; they would likely complain that their cloud was too hard, their wings too tight, or that St. Peter asked too many questions when they entered the Pearly Gates. They have a natural proclivity for finding the worst in any situation, are expert of immediately deducing the problems inherent to a proposed action, and identify quickly where and how a plan will fail once enacted. Over time, they can erode not only pride, but also create a doubt in the steadies' collective consciousness about how strong the organization **really** is, which in turn causes this middle majority to question the organization in general and the physician leader specifically relative to competence and direction. Furthermore, the superstars, who want to be part of a successful team positioned and dedicated to growth and development, will tire of the perpetual and unabated negativity, and eventually seek employment at an organization with a more positive perspective.

To ensure that a positive posture of communication is positioned as a daily expectation, the physician leader should implement a series of house rules for all staff members. These house rules can be posted, or as is the case at many healthcare organizations, printed on the back of the employee's name badge to signal clearly that they are not only job expectations, but work requisites.

- Do not raise a problem unless you are ready to propose at least two solutions.
- When you make a suggestion and suggest a solution to a problem, make sure that the solution is realistic in scope and capable of being implemented readily without undue expense of time, energy, or other precious resources.
- Noise annoys; keep personal problems and opinions away from the patient and visitors, and preferably, away from the hospital.
- Anytime is a good time to ask for help, especially if you feel overwhelmed.

These precepts can prevent the steadies from falling into the Niagara of negativity promoted by the nonplayers while conveying clearly the expectations for work performance beyond the specter of the job description to the nonplayers. It also reflects standards which the superstar already exemplifies, which not only reinforces their work behavior but also provides additional empowerment, as it encourages them to act as leaders in the workplace in providing assistance to steadies as needed and requested.

Priorities Versus Preferences

All employees have their own notions on what is the most important part of their job and definitely can detail their favorite parts of the job. In some cases, their preferences are in accord and alignment with the organization's need for their work contribution, and thus a fusion exists with their strengths and interests as the organization moves forward. However, the organization will invariably expect more from an employee than just their personal favorite parts of their job, and as a result, nonplayers and some steadies can be justly evaluated poorly due to not doing **the whole job**.

The physician leader needs to constantly calibrate performance based on the priorities of the organization, namely

- **The needs, expectations, and demands of the customer:** This can include the basic reason why the customer exists relative to the organization, as well as new trends, emerging demands for new services, and the often-overlooked but ultimately important **human touch** always sought and constantly evaluated by the customer. In essence it is the organization taking good care of business vis-a-vis their customer that is the most important evaluator in the process.

- **The goals, objectives, and strategy of the organization:** The organization's original charter is as important as its current mission statement in this regard and often can be concordant. For example, many metropolitan hospitals on the East Coast were opened in the late 1890s and forwarded a charter of using all of their organizational strengths—mental and physical—in the pursuit of excellence in the interest of taking care of their neighbors who were in pain and need. Newark Beth Israel Medical Center, opened in 1899 with a charter statement which embraces this tenet fully, now has over 4400 employees across the largest medical campus in the nation's most densely populated state, New Jersey. Its strategy is still centered on its original charter, and despite myriad changes in medical technology, constant restructuring of nonprofit healthcare finance, and varied eras of change and competition in urban health care, the mission remains the same and each employee's second priority—next to taking care of the patient, as per our first standard above—is supporting the organization's almost sacred charter in taking care of the healthcare needs of the state's largest city.

- **The operational imperatives of the work team:** It is the responsibility of the team leader to ascertain the best work flow and assignment of responsibility to each team member in a manner that both utilizes the individual talent of the employee while garnering maximum return on investment relative to the organization's goal. The sometimes elusive **value proposition** of each employee should be appraised by the physician leader and then used in concert with the whole team to provide maximum contribution to the organization's mission.

- **The individual daily action of the employee:** The duality of the employee's action being the fourth priority is the epitome of a double-edged sword proposition. On one hand, the employee should think of the patient's needs, the organization's mission and contribution to the team's success progressively—in taking care of those three objectives, he/she is in essence taking care of himself/herself. On the other hand, if the employee does not meet the demands of all three of these dimensions, the entire operation can fail in some regard, as the employee represents the nuclear strength of the organization. Accordingly, the strategic leader should use all four dimensions in this sequence in all communications:

  1. What is the best action needed individually to meet a customer's expectation?
  2. What course of action would reflect the best credit on the organization's mission?
  3. How does this particular employee make the optimum contribution to the team?
  4. How do I best play to the strength(s) of this employee, based on the three factors above?

Inspiration Versus Obligation

Motivation is a topic which has filled tomes of management literature since people tried to figure out what made Adam bite that apple. From Maslow to the late Steven Covey, the topic has fascinated psychologists in general and management scholars alike. This PACT Factor can easily be interpreted as another attempt to gild the basic concept of **the carrot** (inspiration) and **the stick** (obligation), but the idea here is more rudimentary than grandiloquent. Relative to accountability, the mediocre performer works from a reactionary perspective and has limited opportunity for personal growth and professional development. Their sole motivation at work is a paycheck, which in turn pays for obligations such as rent, food and transportation, and maybe a disposable income item or two which make them forget that they are bored in their job and essentially unfulfilled professionally.

The primary component in this couplet, inspiration relates to four concepts which can be utilized positively by the strategic leader with their staff and indeed are likely part of the work orientation of the physician leaders themselves.

> **Work interest:** If an employee enjoys about 70% of their job responsibilities, they will contend with the 30% that is less interesting and engaging. If that quotient is higher, the employee will become even more motivated. If it is less, the employee's performance will either erode, as would likely be the case with a steady, or the employee will seek new employment, as would be the case with the superstar (Figure 2–5).

> **Knowledge:** Many clinical specialists in health care found their way into their profession based on a passion for science that was apparent early in life. Likewise, many human resource professionals in health care consider themselves not only **people persons**, but individuals with a deep interest in **figuring out what makes certain people tick**—a good interest base for someone who interviews job candidates.

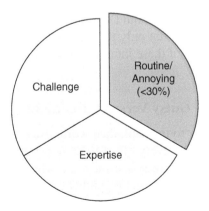

FIGURE 2–5. Work interest.

However, these established interests and passions must be augmented with formal education and training to fully develop their acumen in their profession. Knowledge must be an accountability shared by leader and staff member alike as a continuous and constantly evolving process.

Intrinsic drive: Put simply, the employee must **want to** do the job. For a team of high potential students at Asbury Park High School, to cite an example of the work of the Stevens Healthcare Educational Partnership, the drive to attain a good career through the opportunity to go to a good college and have a career in health care is the drive for this cadre to come to SAT prep classes in the middle of July. For a team of physicians at nearby Monmouth Medical Center, the drive is derived from wanting to see how much healing can be accomplished with the resources at hand in a hospital which was opened nearly 150 years ago as a railroad workers' hospice. This facet of motivation might be nebulous in definition, but apparent immediately by just observing the intensity of work demonstrated by a particular staff member. And among all four of these tenets, it is probably the one that sparks performance in the other three tenets and therefore which must be brought to the workplace from Day 1 by the employee.

Innate ability: This factor is centered on the employee's ability to be able to do the job—the **can do** element which can vary widely among performers, even in the same job category. The lexicon of professional athletics and the world of music is replete with stories of individuals who were born with talent considered average in comparison to their peers, but was maximized by outsized innate drive, attainment of more knowledge than their competitors, and a work interest that was close to the 100% level.

The physician leader should evaluate each employee and provide guidance and support not only through communication, but action in accordance with all of these interdependent and synergistic tenets.

Gutsy Versus Gasconade

If eyes are the window to the soul, then words are the key to action. Physician leaders must make every effort to demonstrate that their words do have meaning, and in essence, that they say what they mean and mean what they say. In a world that seems synthetic with mass media and Internet communication seeming more insouciant and dissonant every day, a leader who makes the tough calls exhibits the small decencies and knows that there is no such thing as **conditional integrity** cuts a strong swath among their staff and goes a long way to establishing trust.

While no tenet of human behavior can be considered an **absolute**, the establishment and maintenance of trust might be the one exception. If an individual trusts a friend, coworker, or family member and then witnesses an episode in which they feel that trust was compromised—that is, they were **burned** by the person they trusted, either perceptually or in reality—it will be difficult if not impossible for the offending party to completely regain the complete trust of the offended party. Try as they might, there will always be a shadow of doubt and 100% trust will never be recovered.

To establish trust among their charges, physician leaders should demonstrate not only through words but more importantly, through actions resonant of the bromide **talk is cheap**, five essential values that are held in high esteem by right-thinking staff (read: the superstars and steadies). While values are typically classified as verbs, consider the application of these values in a predicate sense—that is, as verbs (Figure 2–6). For example, either physician leaders **value** integrity or they do not. The physician leaders **value** the attainment of meaningful, purposeful knowledge in the workplace as a common objective or they do not.

Decency: The desire to do the right thing in every given situation

Fortitude: Fighting the good fight

Industry: Working hard and equally important, working smart

Integrity: Unfailingly honest and forthright in every communication

Knowledge: Striving to learn something new every day at every opportunity

In addition to being leadership standards, these five values can be communication guides that should be the norms in a progressive workplace. As a refreshing contrast to the bloviating and obfuscation of the nonplayers, these standards represent the most appropriate way to communicate in a progressive workplace.

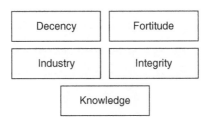

FIGURE 2–6.   Defining values of a superstar—DFIIK Formula.

SUMMARY

This chapter provides not only standards but strategies which are easily applied to any workplace. Used concordantly with the other strategic communication and leadership strategies in this book, immediate positive outcomes can be realized among the most significant resource of an organization—the employees—who are the driving force and centric foundation of any progressive organization.

PRACTICAL RESOURCE—CHAPTER II:
Countering Nonplayer Excuses

This practical resource provides some field-proven, readily applicable communication strategies to diminish the negative impact of the nonplayer.

LINE 1: YOU DON'T LIKE ME!

Basic Psychology

A favorite nonplayer strategy is to make all work issues personal. When nonplayers are asked to work harder for the renewed organization, they will try to make it a personal issue between the manager and themselves, not a business imperative. Because most managers want to be liked, they fall prey to this particular tactic. It is more important to be understood and respected, however, than liked and accepted.

Recommended Response

It is not an issue of whether I like you personally or not; what I don't like is your performance, and here are two examples to discuss.

At this point, the manager should present, honestly and accurately, two examples of how the nonplayer is ineffective, incompetent, or inadequate.

LINE 2: IF MY PERFORMANCE IS SO BAD, MAYBE I SHOULD QUIT.

Basic Psychology

The nonplayer recognizes that most managers want to help and assist their employees. Nonplayers therefore believe that in the opinion of a manager the greatest failure can be the resignation of an employee.

Recommended Response

If you've decided that you cannot meet the performance expectations that we now hold for all individuals in your position, I will accept your resignation immediately.

This reply shifts the accountability for the nonplayer's future actions from the manager to the nonplayer. By using the pronoun *we*, the personal issue is removed and replaced by the business issue of whether the nonplayer wants to meet the new organization's requirements. In most cases, the nonplayer will not resign, but in some happy instances they may. Under no circumstances should a resigning nonplayer be rehired. In the majority of cases, this will be the last time that the nonplayer plays this particular game.

LINE 3: I'VE GOT A PROBLEM WITH THAT.

Basic Psychology

As discussed previously, this is a favorite trick of the nonplayer. The non-player's intent is to force the manager to wrestle with a problem that cannot be solved, thus losing credibility with the nonplayer, as well as the rest of the staff.

Recommended Response

A solution to your problem would be more useful and a better use of our time. Can you provide one?

Again, this places accountability for the problem solving where it should be—with the individual employee. If this employee can recognize a problem, certainly he/she is intelligent enough to suggest a solution.

LINE 4: WE TRIED THAT BEFORE BUT IT DIDN'T WORK.

Basic Psychology

Here the nonplayer is focusing on the old organizational structure and attempting to dredge up unfortunate past history.

Recommended Response

Tell me what will work now.

This forces the nonplayer to deal with the here and now of the renewed organization; it also sets a precedent that the past is only useful if it is positive.

LINE 5: IF IT AIN'T BROKE, DON'T FIX IT.

Basic Psychology

A nonplayer is threatened with anything that is new and more demanding, as well as unfamiliar. Accordingly, they resist **any** form of change.

Recommended Response

So-and-so just had to downsize because of that type of thinking.

The manager should cite any well-known healthcare organization that was forced to dismiss any number of employees—and unfortunately there are many. This response demonstrates to nonplayers, as well as the other staff, that downsizing of the wrong kind occurs when individuals wait to be acted upon instead of being proactive.

LINE 6: I'M DIFFERENT.

Basic Psychology

Most nonplayers have usually been employed by the organization for a long time. Therefore, they believe that they should be treated especially because of their tenure and experience. Rather than trying to force the nonplayer into uniformity with the rest of their colleagues, the manager should exploit the **differences** of the nonplayer tactfully.

Recommended Response

I would expect more from someone of your experience and tenure.

This again places the burden for positive action and progressive thought on the nonplayer. Because most nonplayers dwell in negativity, this effectively negates the complaint.

LINE 7: IT'S NOT IN MY JOB DESCRIPTION.

Basic Psychology

Most nonplayers can cite their job description completely and use it as an excuse for not assuming new duties. The manager can ask nonplayers to redefine their job description by using a position analysis technique with the help of a human resources specialist.

Recommended Response

All of us recognize that our job descriptions are only 70% of our actual responsibilities. Let's talk about the duties all of us are now expected to perform.

This response sends a strong message to nonplayers that a wider range of responsibilities will be expected of them and that they are part of a cohesive, interdependent unit, not simply individuals entitled to a paycheck for only doing 70% (or less) of their job position's scope. Strict adherence to that description is, in reality, dereliction of duty.

LINE 8: THAT WON'T WORK.

Basic Psychology

Most nonplayers enjoy creating doubt, suspicion, and apprehension in the workplace, which reflects their overall negativity and general dissension with positive work goals.

Recommended Response

What will work?

Once again, the manager must shift the focus from redefining the problem to solving it.

LINE 9: WE'VE ALWAYS DONE IT THAT WAY.

Basic Psychology

The nonplayer loves to dwell in the past.

Recommended Response

There will be more change in health care in the next 2 years than ever before—that way won't get it done anymore.

This recommended response can be followed by a reminder that the organization has just gone through an extensive renewal process to come up with a new, better way of doing business. Either the nonplayer will be part of the solution or he/she will become an ineffective part of the problem—and be treated as such.

LINE 10: SEVERAL OF US THINK THAT.

Basic Psychology

The nonplayer is trying to enlist group support for negativity and contentiousness.

Recommended Response

That's probably just your opinion.

And it probably is. Many managers make the mistake of asking, "Who else believes this?" which plays into the hand of the nonplayer, who then answers, "Well, that's confidential." By stripping the nonplayer of perceived group support, he/she is isolated correctly.

LINE 11: I'M STRESSED!

Basic Psychology

The nonplayer is using stress—a valid feature in the healthcare workplace, especially during reorganization—as an excuse for nonperformance.

Recommended Response

Give me a specific example, or, the patient is the only person owed a stressless existence.

Unless nonplayers can provide a specific example of how they are unduly affected by stress, this again is merely an excuse, not an honest work concern.

LINE 12: I'M NOT COMFORTABLE WITH THAT.

Basic Psychology

The nonplayer is using the issue of job comfort—which could be legitimate under different circumstances—in a nonvalid manner.

Recommended Response

What will make you more comfortable? Or state simply, the patient is the only individual owed comfort.

Once again, the manager must seek to make the complaint specific, work related, and legitimate, or handle it as it probably is—as a sneaky excuse for nonperformance.

LINE 13: THAT'S NOT PROFESSIONAL.

Basic Psychology

Most nonplayers confuse professionalism with their intention to do things the way they want to do them.

Recommended Response

Define professionalism for us.

Nonplayers will have difficulty doing this and will merely revert to reciting how they have been victimized by the new system. Once again, by using **we** or **us** instead of **me** or **I**, the manager can negate this nonplayer tactic.

LINE 14: THIS ORGANIZATION DOES NOT PROVIDE QUALITY SERVICE.

Basic Psychology

With the emphasis over the past several years in the healthcare environment placed on an array of quality service initiatives, the nonplayer can suggest that the reason for their lackluster performance is found in a lack of commitment to healthcare quality on the part of the organization. In essence, the contention is that the organization, not the nonplayer, is the entity which is not performing at a high level.

Recommended Response

If what we're planning and undertaking currently takes care of the patient in a more effective manner, how it is not quality driven in intent?

The nonplayer must now innovate a better approach to performance or simply desist in offering this excuse routinely when pressed for improved individual performance.

LINE 15: COMMUNICATION IS A BIG PROBLEM!

Basic Psychology

As discussed throughout this book, communication is a complex process and therefore can be cited by a nonplayer as a problem at almost every conceivable juncture.

Recommended Response

If we tell you what to do, when to do it, and how to do it, and we communicate to you in a style that is understandable, we have not failed you, you have failed us.

The power of pronouns and action orientation is used progressively in this response.

LINE 16: YOU WON'T LET ME TALK.

Basic Psychology

The nonplayer is suggesting that the manager is trying to prevent him/her from speaking, when really the manager is probably trying to curtail complaining.

Recommended Response

We'll let you talk. We just don't need to hear constant complaining and whining.

The best solution, obviously, is to be honest and direct in calling the nonplayer's behavior exactly what it is—unnecessary complaining.

LINE 17: YOU'RE RACIST (SEXIST, ETC.).

Basic Psychology

The nonplayer is maliciously trying to interject illegalities into the work discussion.

Recommended Response

If you truly believe that I treat you differently from other individuals in your work position, we will postpone this discussion until I can get a third party to join us.

Under no condition should managers try to handle this without the assistance of at least their manager, if not the CEO. At this point, the nonplayer should prove discrimination by concrete examples or be properly documented for slandering the manager.

LINE 18: WE DON'T TAKE CARE OF THE PATIENT ANYMORE.

Basic Psychology

The nonplayer is trying to use patient focus to further self-interest.

Recommended Response

The entire purpose of the renewed organization is to take better care of the customer/patient, as most of us understand.

By citing the renewal process, and in the absence of specific examples by the nonplayer, the manager additionally enlists the unspoken support of all staff for the renewed organization.

LINE 19: ALL OF US ARE SCARED.

Basic Psychology

Once again, the nonplayer is trying to derail organizational renewal by suggesting that everyone is afraid of the process.

Recommended Response

On the contrary, I think you're wrong, because it is quite apparent to me that most of the staff is committed to the renewed organization, as evidenced by their recent actions and behavior.

Once again, the manager is specifying that this complaint is centered on the nonplayer, not on the work group.

LINE 20: I LIKED IT BETTER IN THE PAST.

Basic Psychology

Apparently, the nonplayer, who now has more responsibilities, would love to return to the past. Doing so is inconceivable, unrealistic, and foolhardy.

Recommended Response

As we have discussed over the past several months, a new organization is necessary for the new demands that our patient and our community have for us.

Notice that the emphasis is on patient, community, change, and renewed organizational strength, which is exactly where it should be.

Although the list is not all-inclusive, these 20 excuses are among the more obvious games that the nonplayer plays. By applying common sense and fortitude when using these responses, the nonplayer's effect can be diminished, if not nullified completely as you undertake your physician leadership role.

CHAPTER THREE

A Healthcare Leader's Guide to People Management

As a healthcare or physician leader, no resource is more vital to your department—or, indeed, your organization as a whole—than your human capital. In today's competitive career marketplace, utilizing strong recruitment techniques goes hand in hand with understanding the latest legal policies and labor practices. The process of selecting quality employees requires managers to go through six distinct phases before hiring. Orientation, training, and performance appraising are all activities managers engage in to develop strong employees. Turnover and termination compel managers to continually engage in the hiring and training process. Managers who respond appropriately to office conflict and politics shape a more productive workplace for themselves and their staff members.

MEETING TODAY'S HUMAN RESOURCE DEMANDS

People, in all of their diversity, are essential in healthcare organizations. No one's talents can be wasted in the quest for high performance or greater efficiency. In principle, at least, the following slogans say much about the importance of the human beings that make up today's organizations:

- People are our most important asset.
- It's people who make the difference.
- It's the people who work for us who determine whether our healthcare organization thrives or languishes.

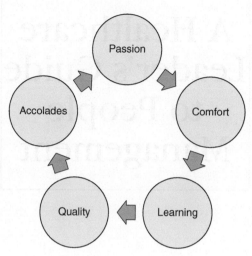

FIGURE 3–1.　Climate components for building staff.

The basic building blocks of any high-performance healthcare organization are talented workers with relevant skills and great enthusiasm for their work. One manager summed up the situation as such: "If you hire the right people ... if you've got the right fit ... then everything will take care of itself." As depicted in Figure 3–1, ensuring that you are doing all that you can to make all of your staff members meet their top potential by playing to their strengths is the starting point for maximizing staff performance.

HUMAN RESOURCE MANAGEMENT

Human resource management (HRM) involves attracting, developing, and maintaining a talented and energetic workforce to support organizational mission, objectives, and strategies. In order for strategies to be well implemented, workers with relevant skills and enthusiasm are needed. The task of human resource management is to make workers available.

- **Attracting** a quality workforce involves human resource planning, recruitment, and selection.
- **Developing** a quality workforce involves employee orientation, training and development, and career planning and development.
- **Maintaining** a quality workforce involves management of employee retention and turnover, performance appraisal, and compensation and benefits.

Additionally, human resource management must be accomplished within the framework of government regulations and laws. All managers are expected to act within the law and follow equal opportunity principles. Failure to do so is not only unjustified in a free society, but it can also be a very expensive mistake resulting in fines and penalties.

The American legal and regulatory environment covers human resource management activities related to discrimination, pay, employment rights, occupational health and safety, retirement, privacy, vocational rehabilitation, and related areas. It is also constantly changing as old laws are modified and new ones are added.

A PRIMER ON THE LAW AND LEADERSHIP

Legal issues in human resource management are continually before the courts. The more prominent among them are frequently in the news. Committed healthcare managers and human resource professionals need to stay informed on the following issues of legal and ethical consequence. There are a myriad of important issues that impact the healthcare work environment every day. In this section, a basic overview is provided to help parse **fact from fiction** with the proviso that anytime is a good time to get an assist from your human resource department when confronted (if not confounded) by a potentially legal situation with a staff member.

Employment discrimination is when someone is denied a job or a job assignment for reasons that are not job relevant. It is against federal law in the United States to discriminate in employment.

An important cornerstone of legal protection for employee rights to fair treatment is found in Title VII of the Civil Rights Act of 1964, as amended by the Equal Employment Opportunity Act (EEOA) of 1972 and the Civil Rights Act of 1991. A working synopsis of important legislative stricture includes

- **Equal employment opportunity (EEO):** The right to employment without regard to race, color, national origin, religion, gender, age, or physical and mental ability. The intent is to ensure all citizens have a right to gain and keep employment based only on their ability to do the job and their performance once on the job.

EEO is federally enforced by the Equal Employment Opportunity Commission (EEOC), which has the power to file civil lawsuits against organizations that do not provide timely resolution of any discrimination charges lodged against them. These laws generally apply to all public and private organizations employing 15 or more people.

Under Title VII, organizations are also expected to show **affirmative action**.

- **Affirmative action** gives preference in hiring and promotion to women and minorities, including veterans, the aged, and the disabled. Affirmative action ensures that women and minorities are represented in the workforce in proportion to their actual availability in their respective labor market area.

- **Affirmative action plans** may also be adopted by or required of organizations to show that they are correcting previous patterns of discriminatory activity and/or are actively preventing its future occurrence.

The pros and cons of affirmative action are debated at both the federal and state levels, and controversies often make the news. Criticisms tend to focus on the use of group membership (eg, female or minority) instead of individual performance in employment decisions. The issues raised include the potential for members of majority populations to claim discrimination. White males, for example, may claim that preferential treatment given to minorities in a particular situation interferes with their individual rights as a claim of **reverse discrimination**.

As a general rule, EEO legal protections do not restrict an employer's right to establish **bona fide occupational qualification (BFOQ)**.

- **Bona fide occupational qualification:** Criteria for employment that can be clearly justified as being related to a person's capacity to perform a job.

The use of bona fide occupational qualifications based on race and color is not allowed under any circumstances; those based on sex, religion, and age are very difficult to support. Years ago, for example, airlines tried to use customer preferences to justify the hiring of only female flight attendants. It didn't work; today men and women serve in this capacity.

In addition to race and gender, which get a lot of attention in the news, other areas of legal protection against discrimination also deserve a manager's concern. Listed below are four examples and brief summaries of their supporting laws. The complexities of these laws would require further research into the context of any possible case to which the laws may be applied.

- **Disabilities:** The Americans with Disabilities Act of 1990 prevents discrimination against people with disabilities. The law forces employers to focus on abilities and what a person can do. Increasingly, persons with disabilities are gaining employment opportunities.

- **Age:** The Age Discrimination in Employment Act of 1967 (amended in 1978 and 1986) protects workers against mandatory retirement ages. Age discrimination occurs when a qualified individual is adversely affected by a job action that replaces him or her with a younger worker.

- **Pregnancy:** The Pregnancy Discrimination Act of 1978 protects female workers from discrimination because of pregnancy. A pregnant employee is protected against termination or adverse job action because of the pregnancy and is entitled to reasonable time off work.

- **Family matters:** The Family and Medical Leave Act of 1993 protects workers who take unpaid leaves for family matters from losing their jobs or employment status. Workers are allowed up to 12 weeks' leave for childbirth, adoption, personal illness, or illness of a family member.

- **Sexual harassment:** Sexual harassment occurs when a person experiences conduct or language of a sexual nature that affects his or her employment situation. According to the EEOC, sexual harassment is behavior that creates a hostile work environment, interferes with their ability to do a job, or interferes with their promotion potential.

- **Equal pay:** The Equal Pay Act of 1963 provides that men and women in the same organization should be paid equally for doing equal work in terms of required skills, responsibilities, and working conditions. However, a lingering issue involving gender disparities in pay involves **comparable worth**, the notion that persons performing jobs of similar importance should be paid at comparable levels. Why should a long-distance truck driver, for example, be paid more than an elementary teacher in a public school? Does it make any difference that the former is a traditionally male occupation and the latter a traditionally female occupation? Advocates of comparable worth argue that such historical disparities are due to gender bias. They would like to have the issue legally resolved.

- **Part-time and temporary workers:** The legal status and employee entitlements of part-time workers and independent contractors are also being debated. In today's era of downsizing, outsourcing, and projects, more and more people in all industries—including health care—are being hired as temporary workers who work under contract to an organization and do not become part of its official workforce. They work only **as needed.** Problems occur when these individuals are engaged regularly by the same organization and become what many now call **perma-temps.** Even though regularly employed by one organization, they work without benefits such as health insurance and pension eligibilities. If they were legally considered employees, these independent contractors would be eligible for benefits, and the implications for their employers would be costly. A number of legal cases are now before the courts seeking resolution of this issue.

- **Labor-management relations:** Union representation for healthcare workers is becoming increasingly common, particularly in larger cities where sizable groups of professionals with similar skills and employment opportunities exist. Nurses of various levels, laboratory technicians, and even office managers can belong to unions. Healthcare labor unions are frequently involved in contract negotiations and unfair employment practices investigations. Labor-management issues and their legal foundations are discussed later in the chapter.

LABOR-MANAGEMENT RELATIONS

Another aspect of human resource management relates to the influence of organized labor. **Labor unions** are organizations to which workers belong that deal with employers on the workers' behalf. Labor unions act as bargaining agents, negotiating legal contracts that affect many aspects of human resource management. Labor contracts typically include the rights and obligations of employees and management with respect to wages, work hours, work rules, seniority, hiring, grievances, and other aspects of employment. The foundation of any labor and management relationship is **collective bargaining**, which is the process of negotiating, administering, and interpreting labor contracts. Labor contracts and the collective bargaining process are governed closely in the United States by a strict legal framework.

- The Wagner Act of 1935 protects employees by recognizing their rights to join unions and engage in union activities.
- The Taft-Hartley Act of 1947 protects employers from unfair labor practices by unions and allows workers to decertify unions.
- The Civil Service Reform Act Title VII of 1978 clarifies the rights of government employees to join and be represented by labor unions.

Often, labor and management are viewed as win-lose adversaries, destined to be in opposition and possessed of certain weapons with which to fight one another. If labor-management relations take this form, a lot of energy on both sides can be expended in a prolonged conflict.

Some believe that this model is, to some extent, giving way to a new and more progressive era of greater cooperation. Fortunately, because most healthcare organizations are nonunion, and the majority of states are **right to work** which means that unions do not control the selection and hiring process, this factor will likely not be prominent in your leadership equation.

HUMAN RESOURCE PROFESSIONALS—KNOW YOUR SUPPORT SYSTEM

Any healthcare organization should at all times have the right people available to do the requisite management support work. Most healthcare human resource departments will provide support in five critical areas.

Recruitment, Selection, and Staffing

- Establish organization standards for new employee selection at both the staff and managerial levels that can be used in both external (new employee) and internal (existing employee) selection.
- Implement recruitment systems that maximize all potential and possible sources for new talent acquisition for all clinical, non-skilled and professional positions.

- Lead targeted searches for high-level positions, as designated by the CEO and COO, to include executive positions and high-demand/low-supply skilled specialist positions.

- Consult as needed and as requested by line managers and directors on the identification of sources for potential candidates for critical positions, and provide specific counsel on the successful recruitment and selection of high-potential new organizational members.

- Lead the processes and programs of new employee orientation to include aiding line managers in specific individual development plan.

- Designate appropriate compensation and benefit packages for incorporation into offer letters and contracts for specified new organizational talent at the exempt compensation level.

Wage and Compensation Administration

- Ensure that all wage levels throughout the organization are competitive in comparison to similar regional organizations and reflective of the job content and professional requisites of the job position.

- Lead effective job analysis and job composition systems to enable efficient performance evaluation, daily management and direction, and clarity of purpose for all employees.

- Maintain job equity standards in all positions across the span of the organization by utilizing appropriate and accurate compensation data, conducting wage and position comparative surveys and other strategies.

- Monitor benefit and compensation programs and packages beyond salary and pay in order to maintain fairness, optimize available payroll and labor budgeted costs, and heighten employee morale and good employee retention.

- Fuse advantageously not only base pay but also cost of living increases, bonuses, incentive pay, and other yearly incentives into tactically insightful performance improvement and quality enhancement programs at the individual, departmental, and organizational levels.

Employee Relations

- Work in concert with the director of organizational development to implement needed education, training and development on key technical, industry and organizational subjects through traditional **in-service**, and other delivery modalities.

- Lead comprehensive and targeted efforts in conjunction with line managers to maintain progressive and positive quality of work life across the panoply of the organization.

- Conduct town hall meetings and other forums that encourage maximum participation by employees to provide input, suggestions, and solution formulation to any and all issues significant to daily work life.

- Act as a moderator for performance improvement discussions when appropriate, and lead initiatives that can help improved communication and action response to significant employee issues at all levels, to include affiliates such as major physician practices and other constituencies in the organization.

- Manage proactively any programs and systems that help maintain the organization's nonunion status and position as an employer of choice in its competitive regional area.

Management Counseling and Support Services

- Assist in the placement, orientation, education, and development of volunteers who while not paid employees must demonstrate the guest relations skills and reflect the professional standards of the organization.

- React immediately and reliably to all requests from managers at all levels of the organization for consultation on performance problems specific to unsatisfactory individual employees and lackluster work groups.

- Lead and manage a staff of human resource and personnel administrative professionals at both the hourly/staff and exempt/ professional levels, as provided and designated by executive leadership in the daily administration of continuous human resource and personnel administration and in response to change/crisis dynamics impacting the organization's human capital.

- Maintain a state-of-the-art IT system that supports all human resource management and personnel administration processes and procedures to include job description, performance evaluation, and compensation data.

Human Resource Management and Personnel Administration Systems

- Compose a dynamic human resource and personnel administration strategic plan for the entire organization by identifying pertinent external dynamics, organizational needs, and growth imperatives relative to the organization's current and emergently needed human capital.

- Implement needed equal employment opportunity, affirmative action and other legally mandated protections, programs and processes comprehensively throughout the organization through education, enforcement, and expedient execution of action as needed.

- Resolve manager-employee conflicts as requested by executive administration or the parties intrinsic to the situation(s) through immediate response, fact finding and direct counseling, and when necessary, with the engagement of legal or other expertise.

- Ensure compliance and constructive response to all relevant national and local existing labor statutes, as well as new mandates that directly impact the organization's workforce and leadership.

- Coordinate and lead all community outreach and local liaison efforts, such as job fairs, educational institution events, and other opportunities to enhance the organization's presence relative to the local and regional communities.

- Contract with needed consultants and other experts economically and pragmatically as needed to continually maximize human resource strength.

PLANNING CONSIDERATIONS FOR YOUR STAFF

- **Strategic human resource planning:** A process of analyzing staffing needs and planning how to satisfy these needs in a way that best serves the organizational mission, objectives, and strategies. The foundations for human resource planning are set by job analysis conducted by human resource professionals with significant input from managers at various levels.

- **Job analysis:** The orderly study of just what is done, when, where, how, why, and by whom in existing or potential new jobs.

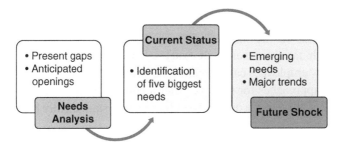

FIGURE 3–2.   Essential checkpoints of HR planning.

Job analysis—which often includes human resource personnel observing and interviewing employees who do a specific job and then collaborating with managers to write a comprehensive description of all that a job entails—provides useful information that can then be used to write and/or update **job descriptions** and **job specifications**, which can then be shared with employees and potential job applicants.

- **Job descriptions:** Written statements of job duties and responsibilities.
- **Job specifications:** Lists of the qualifications—such as formal education, prior work experience, and skill requirements—that should be met by any person hired for or placed in a given job.

The elements in strategic human resource planning are shown in Figure 3–2. The five-step process outlined in the figure begins with a review of organizational mission, objectives, and strategies, which establishes a frame of reference for forecasting human resource needs.

Ultimately, the planning process helps managers identify staffing requirements, assess the existing workforce, and determine what additions or replacements are required to meet future needs. The entire process, of course, must be implemented in a manner consistent with the legal environment.

ATTRACTING A QUALITY WORKFORCE

Attracting and selecting new members of your team can easily spell the difference between success and failure as a healthcare manager. When you select a top performer, you have an individual from whom the entire team can draw inspiration and rely on for steady or stellar performance.

Conversely, when you select an individual who is not a top performer, the negative results can be staggering.

Although far from being an exact science, the process of hiring and selecting new employees can take on some structure, complete with strategies and proven approaches for success. After a human resource plan is prepared, the process of attracting a quality workforce can systematically begin.

- **Recruitment** is a set of activities designed to attract a qualified pool of job applicants to an organization. Emphasis on the word qualified is important.

Effective recruiting should bring employment opportunities to the attention of people whose abilities and skills meet job specifications. The three basic steps in a typical recruitment process are

1. Advertise a job vacancy.
2. Establish preliminary contact with potential job candidates.
3. Perform an initial screening to identify all qualified applicants.

In recruiting potential nursing candidates soon to graduate from a healthcare training school, for example, advertising is done by a hiring hospital by posting short job descriptions in print or on Web sites through the campus placement center. Preliminary contact is made after candidates register for interviews with hospital recruiters on campus. Preliminary interviews typically run 20 to 30 minutes, during which the candidate presents a written resume and briefly explains his or her job qualifications. To further screen the candidates, the hospital recruiter shares interview results and resumes with key decision makers at the hospital. They choose a final pool of candidates to be invited for further interviews during a formal visit to the organization.

Recruitment is certainly one of the most difficult endeavors for the modern-day healthcare manager. The reason for this is the ongoing shortage of qualified personnel in virtually all healthcare positions. This means you must work assiduously toward generating a good roster of candidates and use as many recruitment sources as possible.

External Versus Internal Recruitment

Recruitment can be either internal or external:

- **External recruitment**, in which job candidates are sought from outside the hiring organization. Newspapers, employment agencies, colleges, technical training centers, personal contacts, walk-ins, employee referrals, and even competing healthcare organizations are all sources of external recruits.

- **Internal recruitment** seeks applicants from inside the organization. This involves notifying existing employees of job vacancies. Most healthcare organizations have a procedure for announcing vacancies through newsletters, electronic bulletin boards, and the like. They also rely on managers to recommend high-performing workers as candidates for advancement.

Both recruitment strategies offer potential advantages. External recruiting brings in outsiders with fresh perspectives and provides access to specialized expertise or work experience not otherwise available from insiders. Internal recruitment is usually less expensive and involves people whose performance records are well established. A history of serious internal recruitment can also be encouraging to employees; it shows that one can advance in the organization by working hard and achieving high performance at each point of responsibility.

Recruitment Tactics

Healthcare managers rely on several tried-and-true methods to recruit quality job candidates. Although organizations have specific techniques and resources (consult with your human resource department), the following tactics are all useful:

- **Job fairs:** Whenever possible, try to attend job fairs in your specific technical area. Although many job fair attendees are simply shopping around and aren't interested in immediate employment, collecting resumes and obtaining information on potential candidates is a continuous process for proactive healthcare managers.

- **School liaisons:** Many healthcare professionals maintain contact with the schools they graduated from. Contact the school's placement office or a favorite teacher, and ask whether any up-and-coming talent may be suitable for your open position. School liaisons may also know alumni in the field who may be suitable candidates as well. If you are trying to fill an entry-level position, contact a guidance counselor at a local high school or vocational school and inquire about likely candidates.

- **Employment referral systems:** Most organizations have an employee referral system in which employees refer qualified individuals to human resource for openings in the organization. If your organization does not have an employee referral system or if you work in a small healthcare organization, discuss with your supervisor the possibility of providing a monetary reward to an employee who recommends a candidate for an open position who is subsequently hired.

- **Professional contacts:** Contact former colleagues or institutions and discuss the availability of potential candidates. If you belong to a professional organization, contact a representative within that organization to generate a list of potential candidates.

- **Agencies:** Many healthcare recruiters frown on placement and search agencies because recruitment services are costly and often yield less than satisfactory results. Contact an agency only with the assistance of your human resource department or your immediate supervisor. When you work with an agency, spend as much time as possible with the primary recruiter in developing a list of expectations and revised job descriptions.

- **Advertising:** Employment advertisements in print and online media can be somewhat expensive, and unfortunately they can provide inconsistent results. If you run an advertisement, work with your human resource director and supervisor to craft the advertisement. Make certain the advertisement receives good placement within the newspaper or magazine, has a catchy logo, and contains a three- to five-sentence depiction of the job, the salary range, and the name of a specific contact person. These elements will eliminate people who are simply job shopping or who are not in the salary range established for the position.

- **Team/staff referrals:** Members on your own team may know someone qualified for an open position. However, unless they are asked, your team members may assume you're not interested in their recommendations.

Community-Based Recruitment

Smaller healthcare providers, particularly in rural areas or in distinct neighborhoods (eg, those of large East Coast cities), use community-based recruitment. These institutions write a three- to five-sentence depiction of the open position, the point of contact, and salary range, and make copies on their organization's stationery. They post these copies on bulletin boards in key areas within the community: supermarkets, convenience stores, libraries, community centers, post offices, and places of worship.

When using community-based recruitment, be sure to get permission from the appropriate authority at each posting area. Getting their permission is also an opportunity for you to gain their support and participation in the search effort by reviewing the contents of your notice and discussing any potential applicants they might know among their customers or congregation. The business and religious anchors in the community are typically positive allies in the healthcare recruitment process.

The Selection Process

To avoid the negative aspects of hiring a poor performer, you need to understand the selection process. Selection is the process of choosing from a pool of applicants the person or persons who offer the greatest performance potential. Healthcare managers who successfully master the selection process not only diminish the chance that they have to terminate poor performers or address performance problems, but they also enhance all their management responsibilities by having the luxury of working with well-motivated, talented people.

Figure 3–3 shows the typical steps in the selection process, and the following section explores each step of the selection process in greater detail.

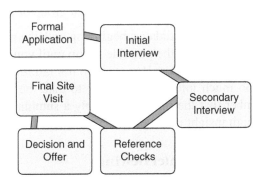

FIGURE 3–3.   Chronology of the selection process.

Reviewing Applications and Resumes

Applicants typically use two important documents to apply for jobs:

- The **application form** declares an individual to be a formal candidate for a job. It documents the applicant's personal history and qualifications. The application should only request information that is directly relevant to the job and the applicant's potential job success.

- The **personal resume** is often included with the job application and should accurately summarize an applicant's special qualifications. As a recruiter and hiring manager, you need to learn how to screen applications and resumes for insights that can help you make good selection decisions.

Your main objective in reviewing resumes is to determine whether the person can do the job. (The interview is where you determine what type of person the candidate is and how they would do the job.) Try to sort the resumes by your criteria, and organize the candidates into three basic categories: unqualified, possible, and probable candidates.

- **Unqualified applicants** simply do not have the quantitative skills established on the job description. For example, they do not have either the required degree or years of experience required.

- **Possible candidates** have the quantitative skills sought and may have additional factors that merit consideration. For example, for the position of staff pharmacist, an individual in the possible category may have all the necessary degrees, including the specific professional accreditation to prepare for state compliance reviews, and a good range of years of professional experience.

- **Probable candidates** are individuals who seem almost perfect for the position. This is typically the smallest group of applicants.

Establish a short list of candidates, beginning with the probable group and including applicants from the possible group until you have approximately seven or fewer candidates. However, do not fall into the seductive trap of reading too much into a resume. Try to take the information at face value; remember that the resume is simply a summary of qualifications, not an in-depth insight into the applicant's personality.

Interviewing

Interviews are extremely important in the selection process because of the information exchange they allow. Thus, a comprehensive interview guide is the resource for this chapter, and this section is provided. The interview is a time when both the job applicant and potential employer can learn a lot about one another. However, interviews are also recognized as potential stumbling blocks in the selection process. To avoid them, keep these general pointers in mind when you conduct a job interview:

- **Plan ahead:** Review the job specifications and job description as well as the candidate's application; allow sufficient time for a complete interview.

- **Create a good interview climate:** Allow sufficient time, choose a quiet place, be friendly and show interest, and always give the candidate your full attention.

- **Conduct a goal-oriented interview:** Know what information you need and get it. Look for creativity, independence, and a high energy level.

- **Avoid questions that may imply discrimination:** Focus all questioning on the job applied for and the candidate's true qualifications for it.

Final Decision to Hire or Reject

The best selection decisions are most likely to be those involving extensive consultation among the manager or team leader, potential coworkers, and human resource staff. The emphasis in selection must always be comprehensive and focus on all aspects of the person's capacity to perform in a given job. Just as a **good fit** can produce long-term advantage, a **bad fit** can be the source of many and perhaps long-term problems. Of course, you should also always remember that you're not seeking the perfect person or perfect match for the position; you're simply seeking the best-qualified person given the criteria for the job. Figure 3–4 provides a quick reference in finalizing a decision on selecting the best possible candidate from a credible pool of interviewed applicants.

DEVELOPING A QUALITY WORKFORCE

When people join any organization, they must **learn the ropes** and become familiar with the way things are done. **Socialization** is the process of influencing the expectations, behavior, and attitudes of a new employee in a way considered desirable by the organization. The intent of socialization in the

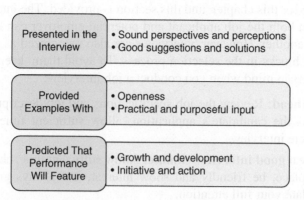

FIGURE 3–4. The best candidate was the one who meets all three of these standards.

human resource management process is to help achieve the best possible fit among the individual, the job, and the organization.

Employee Orientation

Socialization of newcomers begins with orientation. **Orientation** is a set of activities designed to familiarize new employees with their jobs, coworkers, and key aspects of the organization as a whole. This includes clarifying the organizational mission and culture, explaining operating objectives and job expectations, communicating policies and procedures, and identifying key personnel.

The first 6 months of employment are often crucial in determining how well someone is going to perform over the long run. During this time, original expectations are tested, and patterns are set for future relationships between an individual and employer. If orientation is neglected, newcomers are left to fend for themselves during this critical period. On their own or through casual interactions with coworkers, otherwise well-intentioned and capable people may learn inappropriate attitudes and/or behaviors. Good orientation, by contrast, enhances a person's understanding of the organization and adds a sense of common purpose as a member.

Training and Development

Training is a set of activities that provide the opportunity to acquire and improve job-related skills. Training is appropriate and necessary for both new and established employees (particularly those who desire to upgrade or improve their skills to meet changing job requirements).

Training can take many forms:

- **On-the-job training** takes place in the work setting while someone is doing a job.
- **Job rotation** allows people to spend time working in different jobs and thereby expand the range of their job capabilities.
- **Coaching** occurs when an experienced person gives technical advice to someone else. This can happen on a formal basis by supervisors or coworkers. It can also occur more informally in the form of help spontaneously offered in teams.
- **Apprenticeship** is a work assignment as an understudy or assistant to someone who already has the desired job skills. Through this relationship, an apprentice learns a job over time and eventually becomes fully qualified to perform it.
- **Modeling** occurs when someone demonstrates through personal behavior what is expected of others.
- **Mentoring** occurs when new or early career employees are formally assigned as protégés to senior employees who then coach, model, and otherwise assist them to develop job skills and get a good start in their careers.

Performance Appraisal

One of the most difficult responsibilities of a healthcare manager is the assessment and conduct of performance appraisals. Taking qualitative, subjective perceptions of performance and ascribing a quantitative, objective rating is generally a difficult and complex task. This task becomes important specifically as most performance evaluations are tied to the individual staff member's salary and potential salary increases.

Please refer to the performance evaluation resource provided in this book to get a full perspective on this important accountability and to employ a field-proven, ready to implement system to fulfill this responsibility.

Performance appraisals serve two basic purposes in the maintenance of a quality workforce:

- The evaluation purpose is intended to let people know where they stand relative to performance objectives and standards.
- The development purpose is intended to assist in their training and continued personal development.

Performance appraisals should meet the criteria of reliability and validity. To be reliable, the method should consistently yield the same result over time and for different raters. To be valid, it should be unbiased and measure only factors directly relevant to job performance. These criteria are especially important in today's complex legal environment. A manager who hires, fires, or promotes someone is increasingly called upon to defend such actions—sometimes in specific response to lawsuits alleging that the actions were discriminatory. At a minimum, written documentation of performance appraisals and a record of consistent past actions are required to back up any contested evaluations.

Designing and Implementing a Documentation System

Documentation is the process of objectively recording performance and performance levels. Managers and executives at all levels of a healthcare organization rely on documentation to provide proof that accepted standards of performance have been met. Documentation does take time and effort, but without it, the compilation of a comprehensive performance appraisal is next to impossible. Keep the following documentation tips and strategies in mind:

- **Set up a performance documentation logbook.** A simple spiral-bound notebook (or organization-specific log sheets) is all that's necessary to record the dates, significant incidents, and critical contributions for each staff member.

- **Be specific.** General notes like **has a bad attitude** or **never documents well on charts** have little use in preparing a performance appraisal. Whenever possible, note specific, quantifiable details and refer back to established performance objects. And always date any entry in logbooks.

- **Note positive incidents, as well as negative.** Performance appraisals should not be all gloom and doom. Keeping records of what employees do especially well can help your employees recognize their strengths and plan the future paths of their careers.

Finally, realize that whatever form your documentation takes, your professional notes cannot be used or subpoenaed in court. Many healthcare managers fear their notes may be used against them in a court of law. This is not the case, as the only documentation used in a court labor proceeding is the official performance evaluation filed with the healthcare organization. You use your professional notes—not anyone else's.

Use them to increase employees' constructive performance and in turn provide stellar health care to your patients.

Delivering Performance Appraisals

By maintaining detailed, organized documentation, performance appraisals should be relatively easy to write. Sharing appraisals, however, can be another story entirely. The following guidelines can help you effectively deliver appraisals to your employees:

- **Prepare fully for the evaluation.** Ensure you fill out all paperwork correctly and completely. Consider how you want to present the performance evaluation, and simply conduct a review of what you have written on the evaluation.

- **Create an appropriate physical environment for delivering an appraisal.** Sit at your desk, a table, or wherever you are most comfortable; close the door; and avoid interruptions while delivering the evaluation. The occasion should be a private interchange between you and the employee.

- **Provide the employee with a copy of the evaluation.** The employee can use it as a guide, follow the discussion throughout the entire process, and keep the copy as a planning tool for future performance.

- **Manage emotionalism.** If an employee becomes emotional during the evaluation, usually because of a negative reaction, ask whether the employee wants to take a break or reschedule the evaluation. If the employee elects postponement, schedule a follow-up meeting within a week's time and deliver the appraisal fully at that time. If the employee again becomes emotional, either get assistance from your manager or the human resource department, or simply conduct the review in monologue fashion. (Use this last strategy when you suspect the employee is reacting poorly to the performance evaluation as an excuse for poor performance or as a means to avoid the evaluation completely.)

- **Use a direct and objective style.** Use clear terms, state your case objectively, and avoid personalizing the evaluation. Try to stay on an even keel, using emotion only as appropriate. At the same time, feel free to express dissatisfaction to an employee who is not performing acceptably or pride in an employee who is performing at an outstanding level.

- **Use a point-by-point strategy.** Work through the evaluation from beginning to end. Stop frequently to ask whether the employee has any questions or would like elaboration on any part of the information given so far.

- **Set a time limit for the appraisal and stay within it.** For example, an hourly employee may take a half hour to complete a performance appraisal, whereas a skilled worker may need 45 minutes. Try to stay within these parameters and keep that standard for all employees.

- **Give closure.** Ensure that the employee signs the performance-evaluation form and that all questions are answered. Remember, not all employees will be thrilled with their reviews.

Reviewing Group Performance

In addition to individual performance appraisals, many managers conduct team or group performance appraisals. While these appraisals may or may not be required by your specific healthcare organization, group performance appraisals can be worthwhile endeavors. Gathering together as a team to assess the group's strengths and weaknesses, as well as discussing future goals can yield significant results in creating a workplace where employees feel part of a team.

To effectively conduct a group performance appraisal, managers must encourage staff to be direct and candid about their assessment of past performance as a group. Focus the conversation on performance, not on personality-based issues. Avoid referring to the personalities of former managers and other team members. In emphasizing performance, you discover areas for improvement and crystallize specific methods on how to improve performance throughout the department and within individual work roles.

Discussion about what we are doing wrong also helps establish trust. By acknowledging that the department is not perfect and that you as a manager are not perfect, you remind everyone involved that you share the human quality of imperfection. By reviewing mistakes and concentrating on where a problem may exist, your staff will appreciate your commitment to them and therefore feel freer to share their thoughts on areas for improvement.

One way to facilitate a group performance appraisal is to have all team members brainstorm areas for improvement. First, list events or work aspects that need improvement. Then, ask your staff to focus in on things they can control or are doing right relative to the problems or challenges cited. Finally, brainstorm situations and circumstances of which the department has either limited or no control.

In later sessions (or perhaps regular department meetings), you can continue to discuss as a group how the team can become stronger. This could include another exercise on how the team can meet the needs of the patient at an even higher level of quality and effectiveness. Use five basic questions to initiate discussions:

- Where does communication seem to break down?
- When do we operate as a team most efficiently?
- When do we operate as a team least efficiently?
- On a scale of 1 to 10, how would you rate the level of pride we have in our department (1 = no pride, 10 = great pride)?
- What can we do better as a group?

These questions serve to facilitate a group process for discussion of specific areas needing improvement and, more directly, address areas in which the unit can work more strongly as a team.

MAINTAINING A QUALITY WORKFORCE

Attracting and developing a qualified workforce is only a portion of a healthcare manager's responsibilities. For long-term effectiveness, a healthcare workforce must be successfully nurtured and managed. This requires proper attention to such maintenance issues as career planning and development, work-life balance, retention and turnover, and compensation and benefits.

Career Planning and Development

Career planning is the process of systematically matching career goals and individual capabilities with opportunities for their fulfillment. Career planning involves answering such questions as "Who am I?," "Where do I want to go?," and "How do I get there?."

While some suggest that a career should be allowed to progress in a somewhat random but always opportunistic way, others view a career as something to be rationally planned and pursued in a logical step-by-step fashion. In fact, a well-managed career probably includes elements of each. The carefully thought-out plan can point you in a general career direction; an eye for opportunity can fill in the details along the way.

Retention and Turnover

The several steps in the human resource management process both conclude and recycle with the management of promotions, transfers, terminations, layoffs, and retirements. Proactive healthcare managers approach any of these replacement situations as an opportunity to review human resource plans and ensure that the best people are selected to perform the required tasks.

Some replacement decisions shift people between positions within the organization.

- **Promotion** is movement to a higher-level position.
- **Transfer** is movement to a different job at a similar level of responsibility.

Another set of replacement decisions relates to retirement, something many people look forward to—until it is close at hand. Then the prospect of being retired often raises fears and apprehensions. Many organizations offer special counseling and other forms of support for preretirement employees, including advice on company benefits, money management, estate planning, and use of leisure time. Downsizing is sometimes accompanied by special offers of early retirement—that is, retirement before formal retirement age but with special financial incentives.

The most extreme replacement decision involves termination.

- **Termination:** The involuntary and permanent dismissal of an employee. For the person being dismissed, accepting the fact of termination is difficult. The termination notice may come by surprise and without the benefit of advance preparation for either the personal or financial shock.

Compensation and Benefits

When properly designed and implemented, compensation and benefit systems help attract qualified people to the healthcare organization and retain them.

- **Base compensation** is the form of salary or hourly wages that can make the organization a desirable place of employment.

Unless an organization's prevailing wage and salary structure is competitive, attracting and retaining a staff of highly competent workers is difficult. A basic rule of thumb is to study the labor market carefully and pay at least as much as, and perhaps a bit more than, what competitors are offering.

The organization's employee-benefit program also plays a role in attracting and retaining capable workers.

- **Fringe benefits:** The additional nonwage or nonsalary forms of compensation now constitute some 30% or more of a typical worker's earnings. Benefit packages usually include various options on disability protection, health and life insurance, and retirement plans.

Interestingly, the ever-rising cost of fringe benefits, particularly employee medical benefits, is a major worry for healthcare employers. Some are attempting to gain control over healthcare costs by becoming more active in employees' choices of healthcare services and providers. An increasingly common approach overall is flexible benefits, sometimes known as cafeteria benefits, which allow the employee to choose a set of benefits within a certain dollar amount. Employees gain when such plans are better able to meet their needs; employers gain from being more responsive to a wider range of needs in a diverse workforce.

Intangible benefits should also be considered and exploited positively by a healthcare organization. Figure 3–5 provides a vista of these benefits which are seldom used to full advantage and emphasis.

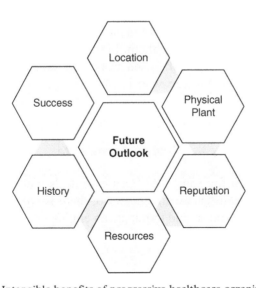

FIGURE 3–5.   Intangible benefits of progressive healthcare organizations.

PROBATION OR TERMINATION

Terminating employees is an unfortunate, vexing but necessary part of being a healthcare manager. Knowing when to fire someone can be as difficult as knowing how. When individual performance has deteriorated to the point of being counterproductive, it is clearly time for separation. In many cases, individuals are actually relieved when terminated because they have become frustrated and ineffective in their work roles.

Do not expect anyone to thank you for terminating them, however, or to admit that it was their fault for being terminated. Terminating an employee is a very difficult undertaking, and this section offers suggestions to make the termination process as painless and productive as possible.

- **Disciplinary probation** is generally acknowledged as a final step before termination. Probation is generally a 3-month process in which poor performers are given the opportunity, usually **one last chance**, to turn performance around to an acceptable level.

Many healthcare managers think that probation is a farce because if the individuals **behave** for 3 months, there is no guarantee that they will perform steadily for the rest of the year. In fact, they generally believe that performance will usually regress.

In many cases, employees who are on probation terminate themselves by securing other employment while on probation, thus saving the headache of having to fire them. In this regard, probation is a worthwhile practice and should be used in conjunction with a performance evaluation for an employee who is likely to be terminated eventually anyway.

When to Terminate

When should you fire someone? Each case deals with unique individual and specific circumstances. In Chapter 6, there is specific guidance and insight into when you should terminate an employee.

SUMMARY

Managing people is the most abstract, qualitative, and challenging component of your role as a leader. By employing the strategies in this chapter and always using the counsel of mentors, senior leadership, and human resource professionals, you will maximize the performance of your staff while optimizing their personal growth and professional development in the workplace.

PRACTICAL RESOURCE—CHAPTER III:
Comprehensive Targeted Selection System

PURPOSE

This resource was specifically prepared for your use in the interviewing and selection process. It provides practical techniques for conducting a thorough, professional interview with targeted behavioral-based questions that are related directly to how we provide health care to our community members. It also contains over close to 200 indicators that will help you make the best possible assessment of the candidate's potential in our organization and in the specific job responsibilities of any open or promotional position.

IMPORTANCE OF SELECTION

Stellar health care begins with the attainment of the best possible human resource talent in all sectors of our organization. Every line manager, director, and executive has no more critical accountability than using their professional expertise and technical knowledge in concert with sound selection techniques to ensure we hire the best possible performers across our organization.

OVERVIEW

The handbook contains three major sections; a practicum on sound interviewing conduct, a battery of 16 sets of interviewing questions (**cues**), interpretative data (**clues**), and a supplemental section with ancillary resources containing management tools such as a guide for conducting exit interviews and a screening guide for phone and initial screening interviews.

Section I: Interviewing Guidelines, Strategies, and Protocol

1. **Preparation and Starting the Interview**
   - Clear your e-mail, mind, and desk space at least 10 minutes prior to the interview.
   - Prepare for the interview:
     - Prepare interview questions using the QCFs to get specific information to match against clues and job descriptions.
     - Use the same questioning strategy with all candidates.
     - Make yourself thoroughly knowledgeable about the candidate prior to the interview and use that base throughout the interview.
   - Always keep your responsibility as an organizational gatekeeper at the forefront of your interviewing strategy and approach. **Keep in mind your role as the organization's representative; to the candidate you are the organization.**
   - Begin the interview with pleasant, professional introductions and appropriate **light conversation** (the weather, first impression of the facility, and a nonsubjective comment from the resume always work).
   - Call the candidate by first name, appropriate title, or preferred nickname (use what/whichever address enhances comfort and flow).
   - Ask the candidate for permission to take notes or merely inform them that you are doing so.
   - Ensure that the candidate is aware of the interview time parameters (and stays within them).
   - Open with the **life story question**.

2. **Conducting the Interview**
   - Respect the candidate's feelings and self-esteem above all else.
   - Always remember that the interview is a public relations tool as well as an assessment of past performance and future potential (most candidates can be our customer patients or know someone who could be).
   - Utilize as many questions as necessary to elicit the necessary responses for key areas of the candidate's background and expertise. Examine and assess candidate's evidence in areas of:
     - Past performance and achievement
     - Work philosophies and beliefs
     - Interview behavior

- Use verbal rejoinders to trigger additional responses in crucial areas; **tell me more…**, **give me another example…**, **what else was involved…**, etc.
- Use nonverbal communication to maintain a steady flow of information in the interview; head nodding, facial/hand gestures, etc.
- Take notes as needed and in a natural sequence, using the response/recall method.
- Describe the position adequately and accurately; question to determine specific candidate's qualifications.
- Don't give excessive encouragement verbally or nonverbally at any point in the interview. Maintain an overall limited emotional profile and avoid emotive reactions.
- Don't use any case study questions, close-ended or illegal questions. Don't use ineffective strategies such as high-pressure/intimidating interviewing.
- Don't wander into EEOC sensitive information unless it is disclosed by the candidate or is a BFOQ (bona fide occupational qualification). Avoid areas such as age, race, marital status, and other sensitive areas.

3. **Maximizing the Interview**
   - Let the candidate do the majority of the talking (80%-90%). Let the candidate do his/her own talking—don't lead or feed the candidate excessively.
   - Listen attentively, accurately, and actively; get the breadth and depth of the information.
   - Interrupt the candidate only when necessary and then with utmost tact and brevity.
   - Downplay excessive negative comments and control excessive rambling by using another question or verbal/nonverbal communication cues.
   - Don't allow the candidate to go so far off track that irrelevant information takes precedence.
   - Ensure that the candidate answers the question at hand completely before moving on to another area. If you don't see the desired characteristic, ask for it specifically; if it is still not apparent, score the interview accordingly.
   - Note how at ease and comfortable the candidate is in the interview question by maintaining a free-flowing communication between the interviewer and candidate.

4. Closing the Interview

- Don't make final appraisal of notes and interview dialogue until the conclusion of the interview. Postpone all final judgment until after the interview. **Avoid the five minute actor factor**.
- Contact good candidates for second interview within 5 days.
- Send marginal and unsuitable candidates' letters of rejection within 2 weeks.
- Keep good resumes on file for at least 1 year.
- Direct the candidate to human resource for explanations on benefits and compensation.
- Give the candidate the opportunity to ask questions but not to conduct another interview.
- Thank the candidate at the conclusion of the interview.

SECTION II: Interviewing Questions and Interpretative Clues

QUAN-COM CATEGORY I: ATTITUDE ORIENTATION

Adaptability: Proven ability to perform well under changing conditions, high stress, and adverse environmental conditions; can relate to a wide variety of personalities and perspectives and absorb new methods with excellent practical results

Accountability: Takes command appropriately in all situations; enterprising, direct and effectively persuasive in all business dealings

Perseverance: Pursues establish work schedule and goals tirelessly into a successful end despite any situational obstacles; willing to go to distance every time

Work ethic: Displays a consistently sound attitude and a positive **can do** approach to all situations; manifests a realistic aura of being capable and ready to perform any tasks that will contribute to the good of the organization

Adaptability:

Proven ability to perform well under changing conditions, high stress, and adverse environmental conditions; can relate to a wide variety of personalities and perspectives and absorb new methods with excellent practical results.

Cues

1. Have you ever lived or worked in a place different or foreign from your hometown?
2. Considering your last or current position, give me some examples of jobs you are asked to do that were not part of the original job description.
3. Detail a unique aspect of your technical area as if I were a potential customer/patient.
4. Tell me about an unusual situation that you had to handle at your last/current position.
5. What radical changes took place at your last job that affected both your role in the organization as well as your daily activities?
6. Tell me about a job situation where you were tasked with handling several things at one time.

Clues

1. Willing to expand on original duties, wants to contribute to learn as much as possible to enhance performance

2. Previous successful adaptations to significant change, that is, new boss, new services, unique business strategies, etc.
3. Consistent past performance under adversity and/or major negative change
4. Demonstrated ability to work with a wide spectrum of people
5. High level of achievement under high stress/pressure
6. Apprehension about a multidimensional/wide-range work role
7. Effective response to change in the interview flow
8. Demonstrated ability to read, react, and readjust effectively
9. Geographic change tempered with success and stability
10. Credible recency, frequency, and intensity of examples

Accountability:
Takes command appropriately in all situations; enterprising, direct and effectively persuasive in all business dealings.

Cues
1. What leadership roles have you held in school/job/community? How did you obtain them?
2. What tactics do you employ to sell a product or products in a customer-patient situation or in other **persuasive opportunities**?
3. How do you open up dialogue when you first meet a new prospective customer/patient?
4. Give me an example of a situation where the customer/patient initially wanted **nothing to do** with your services and/or department.

Clues
1. Holds leadership roles that demonstrate a clear ability to inspire, manage, and lead people; was picked by competitive selection
2. Utilizes a good balance of tact, aggressiveness, and persuasiveness in dealings with others
3. Establishes initial rapport with others (and the interviewer) appropriately, professionally, and with appropriate respect and ultimate impact
4. Credible assertiveness when challenged in the interview forum
5. Stays on message and on point when challenged
6. States his/her case forcefully but tactfully
7. Doesn't hesitate to challenge the norm when necessary by circumstances or need
8. Prohibits aggressiveness and becoming obnoxious, offensive, or pretentious which could diminish impact

9. Doesn't wait to be led or fed in the interview: **Gets off first** and makes point
10. Conveys examples of assuming leadership roles when mandated by situation and circumstance

Perseverance:
Pursues establish work schedule and goals tirelessly into a successful end despite any situational obstacles; willing to go to distance every time.

Cues
1. When confronted with a major obstacle in a business situation, what course of action do you take?
2. Many times the circumstances under which a goal is established change. In this case, would you change your approach or would you change the actual goal itself?
3. Give me an example of a situation at your last/current job that required a lot of persistence/perseverance.
4. Tell me about someone you've worked with who really impressed you with their attitude on the job.

Clues
1. Defines problem, analyzes possible solutions, selects a plan of attack, and resolves the dilemma
2. Provides credible examples of working through a tough problem by fully utilizing all the resources at hand
3. Persistent in answering all cues, even if thrown a curve
4. Willingness to positively attack problems directly, rather than working around them or avoiding them completely
5. Proven ability to function well in a stressful situation/environment
6. Believes in treating all assigned goals and objectives as if they were the most important
7. Appropriately flexible but tenacious in obtaining desired results
8. Doesn't bend to surrounding negativity or ill feelings
9. Can bounce back readily from adversity
10. Doesn't tend to become tunnel-visioned or overtly-hardheaded

Work ethic:
Displays a consistently sound attitude and a positive **can do** approach to all situations; manifests a realistic aura of being capable and ready to perform any tasks that will contribute to the good of the organization.

Cues
1. How do you feel about your current employer?
2. How you feel about your current work situation?
3. Besides yourself, who is the hardest worker at your workplace?
4. How do you feel about the way your career has gone up to present?
5. In your mind, what constitutes a good Jersey work ethic?

Clues
1. Relatively satisfied with accomplishments at present job, but looking for more substantial challenge/career opportunity
2. Feels this position will be a logical **next step**, but takes reasonable pride in accomplishments to date
3. Perceived image stays the same throughout the interview
4. Words chosen to describe sensitive situations are appropriate
5. Realizes the customer/patient is number 1, organization is number 2, the team is number 3, and the individual is number 4 in order of priority in the organization
6. Always willing to give something extra when mandated by the work situation to maintain utmost quality
7. Prides self on professionalism and values it in others; almost intolerant of those who do not put in an equal effort
8. Strives for quality, not just quantity in all endeavors
9. Takes genuine pride in work, company, and self
10. Provides realistic, practical definition of constructive work ethic

QUAN-COM CATEGORY II: PEOPLE SKILLS

Communication: Can express needs and desires effectively to coworkers and superiors in a professional manner; deals tactfully but advantageously with external parties

Energy level: Displays a steady, fast pace in executing assignments, and an innate ability to increase activity to a maximum when necessary; possesses suitable vitality endurance for present and future assignments

Perceptiveness: Has a comprehensive understanding of the human quotient as relates to workplace; the dexterity, and both internal and external interpersonal dealings

Presence/bearing: Creates a positive impression and makes one's presence known in any given situation with favorable results

Communication:

Can express needs and desires effectively to coworkers and superiors in a professional manner; deals tactfully but advantageously with external parties.

Cues

1. Describe the avenues of communication that were available for your use in your last/current job.
2. Detail a procedure or important job component starting with a general overview and tell me about some specifics.
3. Tell me about a coworker who you believe is a great communicator.
4. Tell me about the worst communicator you ever had to work for or worked with.
5. What are 3 or 4 important communication factors in your profession/current job?

Clues

1. Good style of nonverbal communication
2. Nonverbal style is a natural supplement to their verbal style
3. Utilizes syntax, grammar, and tones effectively
4. Seems appropriately natural/comfortable in the interview forum
5. Possesses superior listening skills; readily grasps the **why**, **what**, and **how** of an issue

6. Presents the rationale, method, and outcome of significant achievements
7. Solid questioning procedure when given an opportunity in the interview
8. Uses brevity, gravity, conciseness, and organization in their verbal style
9. Sensitive, succinct, and adroit with sensitive information
10. Doesn't alter or slant objective information
11. Capable of preparing and developing required written/oral reports, as evidenced by past job requirements

Energy level:
Displays a steady, fast pace in executing assignments, and an innate ability to increase activity to a maximum when necessary; possesses suitable vitality endurance for present and future assignments.

Cues
1. What kind of activities do you participate in away from the job?
2. How many hours, on the average, do you spend on the job?
3. How would you rate the enthusiasm of your coworkers at your current position?
4. What particular aspects of your current job get you excited and help spark energy?
5. What job activities sap your energy the most?

Clues
1. Animated in conversation; responds quickly and verbal interaction
2. Discusses situations and experiences positively and looks at the future optimistically
3. Expresses reasonable degree of emotion in the interview
4. Appears more than willing to expand parameters of job scope and amount of work-related activity
5. Maintains a zealous, earnest manner in addressing cues and explaining information; maintains consistent genuine enthusiasm throughout the interview
6. Semblance of an active, balanced lifestyle away from work
7. Energy and enthusiasm lags during the context of the interview
8. Energy and enthusiasm increases when discussing specific aspects of their work role
9. Appears to always work the required amount of hours at a minimum, often works additional hours to ensure excellence
10. Applies energy intelligently; works smart, not just hard

Perceptiveness:

Has a comprehensive understanding of the human quotient as relates to workplace; the dexterity and both internal and external interpersonal dealings.

Cues

1. Give me an example of a tough people problem you had to handle.
2. What would your coworkers say about your people skills?
3. How would your current/past manager characterize your interpersonal strengths?
4. Give me some adjectives that describe your work personality.
5. Tell me about a situation that required some practical application of **people smarts**.

Clues

1. Provides solid examples of dealing with a tough problem successfully while maintaining the best possible interpersonal relations
2. Eminently aware of self-image and how it affects others
3. Stresses people and their intangible qualities as being important in a sincere, genuine manner
4. Appears to be considerate of others in their needs; open-minded to their opinions
5. Can relate to others' viewpoints; adjusts accordingly without vacating personal ideals
6. Consistently stresses other people in the context of the interview
7. Appears to have a good feel for varied personalities; good dexterity in dealing with a wide spectrum of people
8. Enthusiastic when discussing people from past work experience
9. Has a good sense of humor and appropriate warmth style in the interview
10. Does not appear to allow subjective perception to cloud objective facts

Presence/bearing:

Creates a positive impression and makes one's presence known in any given situation with favorable results.

Cues

1. Do you make a conscious effort to convey a certain image?
2. What kind of feedback have you received relative to the way in which you interact with others?

3. Tell me about a customer/organization that has a business image that you can relate to.
4. Who in the public eye has a public image that you admire? Tell me specifically why you admire them and believe their image is positive.
5. Tell me a bit about the culture of your current organization and its relevance to your daily job.

Clues

1. Balances being himself/herself with a solid business style
2. Not overly concerned with presenting a certain image
3. Not a devout advocate of a portrayed organizational style or a rigid manner of external presentation
4. First impression; what would I think of this person if they were dealing with me in a healthcare business relationship
5. Communication style is in sync with their personality
6. Clearly exhibits the attributes of someone who is **comfortable in their own skin**
7. Doesn't project an elitist or aloof presence
8. Projects a genuine, **down-home** natural style
9. Conveys a winning combination of appropriate warmness with dependable professionalism
10. Appears to be a match with our current organizational culture

QUAN-COM CATEGORY III: MANAGERIAL APTITUDE

Creativity: Can innovatively employ both qualitative and quantitative strengths to set action-oriented policy and construct plans that provide result-oriented direction; unafraid to take risks on new programs that can provide improved benefits or more expedient service/ better health care

Delegation: Can assign responsibility and authority in the interest of improving expedience of action; can effectively work through people to accomplish desired ends

Independent judgment: Capable of ascertaining direction and goals utilizing individual talent and ability; basically self-starting, makes judgments and decisions, and executes without undue reliance on others

Planning: Establishes short- and long-range objectives, a progressive course of action for achievement, and an action list of specific tasks; proactive in setting targets and task accomplishment

Creativity:

Can innovatively employ both qualitative and quantitative strengths to set action-oriented policy and construct plans that provide result-oriented direction; unafraid to take risks on new programs that can provide improved benefits or more expedient service/better health care.

Cues

1. What new approaches have you used in your job over the past 6 months?
2. Explain fully a process you were involved with from design through reality.
3. What factors did you consider when you made the decision to _____?
4. Tell me about a new implementation or a new system or procedure that you led at your current job.
5. Tell me about a project where you really had to utilize your imagination.

Clues

1. Routinely looks for and utilizes new approaches which are both proactive and capable of producing better/more results
2. Can expediently but effectively detail a working process in a step-by-step progression to a productive outcome

3. Academic background: type of courses, net yield of education, intensity of study, and ability to apply knowledge base the job needs
4. Heavy reliance on input from others in decision making and plan implementation; constant reliance on mentor figure in thought process
5. Looks for creative openings and resultant opportunity; doesn't have to be pushed into **thinking**
6. Willingly takes risks, even if the decision to do so was unpopular or was considered unorthodox
7. Appears to need a lot of guidance and/or positive reinforcement
8. Takes control of the interview in terms of thought range and idea presentation
9. Displays analytical thinking in explaining processes and procedures
10. Displays conceptual thinking when presenting ideas, opinions, and perceptions
11. Exhibits formidable breadth of knowledge as well as significant depth of analysis

Delegation:
Can assign responsibility and authority in the interest of improving expedience of action; can effectively work through people to accomplish desired ends.

Cues
1. What methods do you use to measure and assign work for others?
2. How do you follow up on work you have assigned to others?
3. Do you think you're a good delegator? Why or why not?
4. When assigning work, what criteria do you consider?
5. Who was the worst boss you have worked for relative to delegation?

Clues
1. Stresses the achievement of others in unit task accomplishment
2. Maintains a set procedure for work measurement, task assignment, and timely completion
3. Stays cognizant of all phases of the operation and the contribution of others relative to outcomes
4. Believes that they are a good delegator and can explain reasons, methods, and examples to support that opinion
5. While believing that they need more development as a delegator, can specify weaknesses constructively and critically

6. Clearly is capable of assembling and managing a team as evidenced by past formats
7. Appears to be able to give our work rather than maintain a high level of ownership
8. Demonstrates perceptiveness relative to subordinate capabilities and limitations
9. Demonstrates innovativeness in utilizing the strengths, talents, and ability of others; consistently plays to their strengths
10. As enabling pastorals to obtain maximum project performance from assign subordinates and peers
11. Maintains responsibility for work **given out**; not a shuffler

Independent judgment:

Capable of ascertaining direction and goals utilizing individual talent and ability; basically self-starting, makes judgments and decisions, and executes without undue reliance on others.

Cues

1. Tell me about an operational problem that you resolved.
2. Tell me about a personnel/human resource/staff problem that you resolved.
3. What programs have you originally conceived and implemented in your career?
4. Have you ever felt as though you've been given more responsibility than you can handle?
5. Tell me about some gambles/risks you've taken in the past that have paid off for you. Why did you take the chance?
6. How do you analyze a situation when pressed for decision? How do you get your data or **the facts**?
7. Would you say you rely more on facts or **vibes**? (Have a candidate defend their choice.)

Clues

1. Utilizes an effective decision mechanism to ensure results are being generated
2. Details resolution of problems that required quick and accurate response
3. Has achieved set goals ahead or on time consistently
4. Responds to questions without undue hesitation with apparent honesty
5. Turnaround time is cited as part of project accomplishment
6. Displays a willingness to get involved with tough situations in the interest of obtaining a positive outcome

7. Can reflect on past experiences and objectively discuss what was achieved and learn
8. Has a proven record of working well independently without alienating peers, subordinates, or superiors
9. Virtually unafraid to take risks if overall result will be favorable to all concerned, notably the customer/patient and the organization
10. Has logical backup reasoning for actions taken in response to challenge/crisis/change

Planning:
Establishes short- and long-range objectives, a progressive course of action for achievement, and an action list of specific tasks; proactive in setting targets and task accomplishment.

Cues
1. What are your career objectives, both short and long range?
2. When you assign a job for you employees to work on, do you let them know exactly what actions they should take or just set a general scope?
3. How do you plan (procedure/team meeting/interview/action plan)?
4. Who is the best planner that you ever worked with?
5. One of this year's hot topics in health care is strategic planning. What does that mean to you pragmatically, and how will it fit into your daily activities in this new job?

Clues
1. Has established a reasonable but challenging plan for career
2. Calibrates work direction and related planning efficiently
3. Routinely analyzes situations and formulates a plan accordingly
4. Conveys future goals in a clear-cut manner and can detail steps which will lead to those goals
5. Well prepared for the interview; knows what he/she wants to present and how it relates to the subject position
6. Seems to chart a logical course of action in attaining goals
7. Capable of explaining plans and the benefit of their implementation
8. Has had to plan daily activities for self and work units in past/current roles
9. Not overly tied to a plan to a point at which changing factors are ignored or optimum performance is sacrificed
10. Delineates data analysis and decision rationale without hesitancy, ambivalence, or retraction

QUAN-COM CATEGORY IV: TEAM ORIENTATION

Cooperation: Highly motivated toward selfless service to coworkers, patients, and organizational goals; looks at tasks as a commitment to others and organizational excellence

Employee-peer relations: Creates and maintains a workplace relationship with assigned subordinates that generates maximum effectiveness and productivity while enhancing motivation and growth; uses human resource as an integral factor in accomplishing goals.

Loyalty/integrity of purpose: Commits to firm contract to work hard for the organization, represents its best interest at all times and toward giving its needs and overall performance top priority; has an intrinsic dedication to the healthcare profession and organizational mission

Technical expertise: Possesses a superlative degree of accrued and formal knowledge of their professional field; able to draw from and specifically apply that knowledge in a proficient manner

Cooperation:

Highly motivated toward selfless service to coworkers, patients, and organizational goals; looks at tasks as a commitment to others and organizational excellence.

Cues

1. In your last or any previous position, did you work as an integral member of a team?
2. What do you foresee as your goals and objectives if you get this job?
3. What do you like about working with people?
4. Tell me about some activities or jobs that have been integral in your life that have required a lot of team orientation.
5. Tell me about a specific situation where you made a wrong decision. How did you remedy the problem?

Clues

1. Total commitment to the goals and objectives of the workgroup and organization
2. Able to act as a resource to others needing technical or peer assistance
3. Willing to help others who are making a solid effort but need assistance
4. Consistently puts group priorities ahead of personal ones
5. Doesn't blame others for mistakes; takes the **bad with the good**

6. Doesn't perceive self as an individual star or as an autonomous performer; stresses the **we** more than the **I**
7. Direct and free in sharing essential information with peers and others
8. Doesn't harbor potentially critical information that is needed by the team and peers
9. Not hesitant in responding to point-blank questions; honest, candid portrayal of past performance
10. Appears genuinely at ease in the interview question; maintains a free-flowing communication between the interviewer and the candidate

Employee-peer relations:

Creates and maintains a workplace relationship with assigned subordinates that generates maximum effectiveness and productivity while enhancing motivation and growth; uses human resource as an integral factor in accomplishing goals.

Cues

1. What types of motivation do you use to help encourage your employees to do their best at their jobs?
2. What kind of relationship do you feel managers should have with his/her staff?
3. Give me an example in your past work experiences where success was predicated on how you effectively trained peers or staff members.
4. Tell me about your leadership philosophy and how people fit into the equation.
5. Who is the best employee that ever worked for you? Tell me what made them so good.
6. Who is the best employee that works for you?

Clues

1. Values the same tenets in employees that the organization values
2. Acutely aware of the need for superior staff members who are superstars in every regard
3. Possesses sound principles of leadership that would have practical use in the new position; wants to do the right thing
4. Possesses sound principles of management; likes to do things right
5. Employees cited as exemplary in past/current jobs have traits that are valued in our organization

6. Fosters a relative system of participatory management when advantageous
7. Can present change openly to employees to a positive end
8. Enthusiastic when discussing personnel from past roles
9. Past roles have produced high productivity, tangible goal results, and low turnover from employees
10. Clearly and concisely delivers work direction to subordinates and staff members

Loyalty/integrity of purpose:
Commits to firm contract to work hard for the organization, represents its best interest at all times, and toward giving its needs and overall performance top priority; has an intrinsic dedication to the healthcare profession and organizational mission.

Cues

1. Why do you work? What are you basic motives in pursuing your career objectives?
2. What are your reasons for leaving (or wanting to leave) your position at _____?
3. What do you think of the people you work with at present?
4. Tell me about your current/past employer. What were some of its best attributes?
5. What kind of commitment you look for from your employer?
6. What kind of commitment do you need from your boss?

Clues

1. Length of time spent in any/each career progression
2. Willingness to speak negatively about other people; **classic badmouthing**
3. Does use tact and brevity/goes overboard in criticizing current/former employer?
4. Overtly disproportionate desire to gain money/social status/personal recognition that is converse to group effort and reward
5. Ego appears to take precedence over all/overall
6. Seeks to always give organization maximum ROI (return on investment) on salary
7. Primary loyalty lies with other things other than family, faith and work; that is, softball career, bowling team, political causes, polemic, etc

8. Seemingly honest, frank, and direct in the interview
9. Not a guppy; loyalty is true fidelity to maximum performance and the organization's goals
10. Past performance/current role reflects the ability to establish a fair but firm relationship with staff members and peers

Technical expertise:

Possesses a superlative degree of accrued and formal knowledge of their professional field; able to draw from and specifically apply that knowledge in a proficient manner.

Cues

1. Explain your range of experience in _____.
2. What do you know about our organization and our healthcare business?
3. How do you keep up with all the new innovations in our/your field?
4. Give me an example of a work situation where your technical knowledge enabled success.
5. Give me an example of a customer-patient situation where your technical knowledge enabled success.

Clues

1. Prior experience in high-stress situations where the customer-patient service is paramount concern
2. Credible range of practical knowledge of subject fields, as evidenced by all indicators
3. Proficient at technical terms
4. Does not use technical terms as code or camouflage that would create unnecessary complexity
5. Good quality technical questions asked were given an opportunity in the interview forum
6. Expresses an interest in learning more about specific area of health care or the business operation
7. Strives to keep abreast of newest trends in field through coursework, reading, professional seminars, etc
8. Active affiliation and participation in recognized professional organizations
9. Attainment of certain specific certifications, degrees, credentials, or related notoriety
10. Can explain technical concepts and processes, so nonrelated personnel can understand and utilize

SECTION III: Screening Interview Tool

The following 6 questions can be used over the phone or in a quick interview (10-15-minute sequence), such as those conducted at a job fair.

1. **Working together:** Tell me about the best team you were ever a part of, including the mission of the team and some of the best members of that team.
2. **Excellence:** What are 2 or 3 projects or programs that you led/ worked on that you are particularly proud of, and what lessons did you learn from them that you could apply at our organization?
3. **Customer service:** What kind of things should a healthcare organization do to really get a good reputation/excellent **word of mouth** exposure in a community?
4. **Accountability:** What are the 3 to 5 biggest responsibilities in your job?
5. **Respect:** What are the worst things an organization can do to diminish respect in the workplace and/or with their customer/patients?
6. **Enthusiasm:** What components of your current/last job really got you excited about going to work every day?

CHAPTER FOUR

Dealing With Politics, Problems, and Process

THE MIASMA OF POLITICS

Unfortunately, as you exercise your talents as a healthcare or physician leader, your patience will likely be tested by overtly political behavior or at least the annoyance of the day-to-day dealings of **office politics**. It is important that healthcare managers avoid political quagmires in the workplace in the interest of providing stellar, progressive services to patients and to the healthcare organization.

Office politics causes several significant problems for the healthcare manager and the healthcare organization as a whole.

- **Politics inhibits productivity.** Generally speaking, workers are not particularly motivated to perform well for individuals who are more politics-minded than performance-minded. A great deal of time is spent avoiding power plays and preparing for counteractions. Consequently, productivity suffers, and worst of all the patient is deprived of receiving the full range of services the healthcare organization is capable of providing.

- **Politics stifles creativity.** Because politics can promote paranoia, team members may be reluctant to share new ideas or work in a group process that encourages creativity or innovation. As a result, staff growth and development are compromised or top performers relocate to a less political or, better yet, nonpolitical environment. Again, the patient and the organization suffer.

- **Politics cripples teamwork.** Individuals who are suspicious of each other and have limited respect for each other end up resenting one another and avoiding open communication. Politics destroys allegiance and loyalty among team members and the overall objective of the team or organization. Group morale begins to diminish until finally individual employee motivation begins to erode.

- **Overt negative politics alters communication.** Overt negative politics includes altered messages, altered presentation of messages, or flat-out noncommunication in certain situations. Politics often begin after a third party enters the picture, creating an unbalanced dynamic and opportunity for two people to discuss a third person—often in an uncomplimentary manner.

Signs of Overtly Political Behavior

Whenever a premium is placed on politics as opposed to performance in the healthcare environment, the team or department finds itself at risk of falling apart—or at least beginning to be much less productive. Five basic indicators that can signal overtly political behavior include

- **Double-talk:** Individuals who tell one story to one person and an entirely different story to another are double-talkers. Their motives may be to cover the bases on a particular issue, deliberately create disharmony, or simply try to pit two people against each other.

- **Backstabbing:** Backstabbers overtly pledge allegiance to you and your ideas but covertly downplay them and insult your intelligence.

- **Power mongering:** Power mongers try to control everything. These individuals are also called turf protectors or empire builders because they often use resources and territory as the principal focus of their subversive efforts. As a healthcare manager, you may fall prey to a power monger's claim of being in charge of something that in fact he or she has no control of.

- **Victim's role:** Some individuals claim that the organization is out to get them and that you had better watch yourself. People with this mindset are more interested in their own survival than in assisting fellow workers through the healthcare mission.

- **Game playing:** Game players use phony behavior in trying to engender support. They play games with fellow staff as well.

Dealing With Overtly Political Behavior

As a physician leader, what are the best strategies for dealing with politics? Whether the politician is a member of your staff or a colleague, these five strategies may be useful:

- **Avoidance** is easy. Simply try to stay out of the way of political behavior whenever possible. If avoidance is not feasible on a daily basis, keep all contact on a business level and discuss only business issues. If someone tries invariably to shift the focus to a politically oriented level, firmly return them to the issue at hand. Remember that your primary managerial responsibility is to bolster staff motivation and productivity while contributing to your facility's goal of high-quality patient care.

- **Confront the person** and let her know that you are aware of her political intent. For example, if you are asked a loaded question, simply counter by asking another question such as, "Why are you asking me that?" You risk incurring wrath, but you at least discourage overtly political behavior.

- **Disclosure and support** works if the troublesome individual is someone on the management team or someone who reports to your own manager. Simply present evidence of the political behavior to your supervisor, without judgment or opinion. Use objective reporting. For instance, "You know, a funny thing happened the other day. I was talking to (name), who seemed persistent in wanting to discuss (topic)." This approach indicates your apprehension in dealing with this individual and signals your need for specific assistance.

- With **direct input** from your own boss, you can actively enlist support. Simply tell your boss—likely a seasoned executive who has dealt with similar games and gambits—about the problem, review the evidence, and ask directly for assistance: "What would you do if you had this situation?" (If you perceive your boss to exhibit excessively political behavior, you may want to request the help of another mentor within the organization in dealing with this behavior.)

- **Gather documentation** as evidence of political behavior by colleagues or staff. The more examples you collect, the better case you can make for termination (if the person is staff) or for limited contact (if the source is a colleague). Record evidence or examples of notable political behavior, and be sure to handle reports tactfully.

RECOGNIZING INTRADEPARTMENTAL CONFLICT

Despite a healthcare manager's best efforts to establish trust throughout his/her work group and to avoid potential conflict, human nature unfortunately creates occasions for intradepartmental conflict. **Intradepartmental conflict** is any conflict that takes place within a single department or work group.

Initially, intradepartmental conflict takes place on an interpersonal basis. Interpersonal conflict, particularly within a work group, is potentially the most damaging type of problem a healthcare manager can deal with. If interpersonal conflict exists within a department and is not abated and resolved correctly, it will have drastic negative consequences for the entire department—even implosion.

Numerous indicators signal intradepartmental conflict. Use your instincts and observations to examine the conflict in a cause-and-effect fashion. Following is a list of potential symptoms, causes, and effects on your department:

- **Anger:** Interpersonal adversity, loss of temper, lack of patience, or flat-out confrontational behavior may all be exhibited in certain kinds of interpersonal conflict.

- **Avoidance:** When an individual declines to work with someone or simply avoids contact with that person, work may not be done and the team processes may be compromised. Avoidance is more subtle than anger and often more common.

- **Blame:** One individual may claim another person is entirely responsible for a mistake. Often the person blaming is attempting to cover for his/her own inability or failure to perform. Blaming creates hostility among team members and betrays basic trust and pride in the organization.

- **Excuse making:** One individual uses another's behavior as a reason for not performing a particular task. The individual may focus specifically on a personality nuance as being the problem that gets in the way of accomplishment. Another form of making excuses is to rationalize the negative behavior of others.

- **Isolation and fragmentation:** Certain team members may exclude one or more players because of personality conflict. Isolation jeopardizes the group participation process, and ultimately, one or more individuals may withdraw the resources needed to get a job done. Extreme isolation may lead workers to organize into factions. This fragmentation can become particularly detrimental in any group process, especially one that requires quick, efficient response.

- **Confrontation:** Argumentative personality types use intimidation and confrontation to disrupt process, waste time, and demoralize others.

- **Criticism:** Continuous nit-picking severely diminishes morale. Ironically, others often respond to constant criticism by becoming defensive and in turn critical of the chronic criticizer.

- **Erosion of performance:** The quality and efficiency of work diminishes, resulting in ill feelings and costly overtime. Some staff begin to look for another workplace if the situation is not corrected by the manager.

- **Regression:** A performance continues to erode, worker may do less and less, bringing work process to a grinding halt. In an era in which health care must be progressive, every employee's performance must contribute to its maximum potential.

RESOLVING INTRADEPARTMENTAL CONFLICT

Many organizations have recommended approaches to dealing with interdepartmental conflict. As you gain more experience as a manager and see what does (and doesn't) work, you're sure to develop your own ways of resolving disagreements between staff members. The following 6-step process can adapt well to a multitude of situations and organizationally recommended processes:

1. **Go on a fact-finding mission.** Begin any effort to resolve intradepartmental conflict by performing thorough fact-finding every step of the way. **Fact-finding** is the process of collecting information from all involved parties before arriving at a decision. For example, when an intradepartmental conflict takes place between two individuals, you may want to investigate by discussing the situation with both parties separately and by asking them the same two questions: what they think the problem and root cause may be, and how the

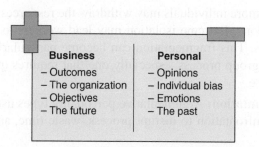

Business	Personal
– Outcomes	– Opinions
– The organization	– Individual bias
– Objectives	– Emotions
– The future	– The past

FIGURE 4–1.   Business versus personal issues in a conflict situation.

situation can be resolved. At that point, bring both parties together, present both ideas for resolution, and once again state your optimism for correction as well as your refusal to tolerate further interpersonal conflict.

2. **Separate issues into two categories.** First identify business-related attributes of the problem—business outcomes, performance dimensions, and technical areas. Then list personal issues that may bear on the conflict (Figure 4–1). Review this information completely with the involved party and reach consensus on the facts of the issues. If no one acknowledges the facts, you may have to state more directly your belief in their validity and supplement that statement with the pledge that you will not accept this behavior any longer.

3. **Move the discussion to performance.** Focus specifically on the business effects from the conflict. Cite work that is not being done; explain how the employee's (or group's) behavior affects other department members and how this behavior interferes with others' getting their jobs done. Discuss further how this behavior affects other departments and, most important, patients.

4. **Ask why this behavior has taken place and how it might be corrected.** Try to get to the bottom of what the parties believe is contributing to the problem and how the cause can be alleviated. Following this discussion, present your own ideas on why the problem exists; however, spend most of your discussion on how the problem must be remedied.

5. **State clearly, concisely, and resolutely your expectations, standards, and policies for future action.** Explain what you accept as satisfactory behavior and what you consider poor performance or

interpersonal conflict. Future actions may include probation or other disciplinary action, including termination.

6. **Express your confidence that the situation will be corrected, and ask whether particular assistance is needed to do so.** Try to strike a delicate balance between expressing optimism that the situation can be corrected and underscoring the fact that continued poor performance and intradepartmental conflict will not be tolerated under any conditions. Interpersonal conflict is complex and can hinder progressive action. As a manager, you must deal with it resolutely and in a timely fashion so that the majority of your department is not adversely affected.

LEADING THROUGH CONFLICT, CHANGE, AND CRISIS

Invariably, healthcare managers must make the tough calls. This includes taking disciplinary action (including terminating employees and putting employees on probation), mediating conflict, dealing with internal customers, and an array of other potentially volatile situations. No matter what your technical background might be or which department you work in, inevitably you will have to manage tough situations—dissatisfied or even hostile customer/patients, for example. Because these situations erupt immediately, you must be prepared with techniques to manage them.

This section deals directly and practically with an assortment of problems a newly appointed healthcare manager can encounter. Although no one solution meets all problems, the information in this chapter should prove to be a useful guide as you attempt to manage those **gray areas** inherent to tough situations. By adopting the strategies most suitable to your management style and work environment, you will take a proactive approach to problem solving and conflict management.

Next, the section will discuss the symptoms of conflict within the workplace and pragmatic ways of resolving conflict among employees. Conflict resolution involves use of fact-finding processes, so an adaptable approach to fact-finding and a strategy for implementing conflict resolution systems into your responsibilities will be offered. Some insight will be provided on counseling employees and resolving conflict in one-on-one counseling situations.

Because probation and termination are unpleasant realities of management responsibilities, these issues will be addressed specifically when and how to fire someone. The section will conclude with a discussion on how to resolve customer/patient complaints successfully and efficiently. Source material is drawn from some of the most challenging complaints from physicians and union employees.

THE ESTABLISHMENT OF TRUST

Regardless of the size of a healthcare work group, there are two elements that cannot be fully regained if lost. One is trust, defined here as the sense of integrity that exists between employees and their supervisor. If trust is lost or diminished through action and negative consequence, it is unlikely that it can be regained at its original level. The other element, pride, is defined here as a sense of allegiance and high esteem that pervades the work group. Both trust and pride are valued commodities that link the supervisor and the individual employee. Trust, however, is the overriding motivator.

This section will discuss ways to establish trust in your work group. It is essential that you embrace these guidelines and try to apply them to your everyday activities. Unless employees have trust in your leadership ability, they may not be motivated to follow even the clearest direction. The consequence is that time will be wasted unnecessarily by challenges to your authority or misguided questioning of your decisions.

You begin to establish trust on day 1 of your tenure as a manager. As alluded to briefly at the outset of this chapter, loss of trust usually results in the breakdown of group harmony and productivity; ultimately, this loss of trust could lead to a manager's termination (Figure 4–2). Many new managers are filling vacancies created by predecessors who in failing to elicit trust from staff failed ultimately to elicit high-quality outputs. In the long run, the establishment of trust could be your most important asset as a healthcare manager.

Ensuring Clear Communication

Communication is the cornerstone for establishment of trust. If you demonstrate a clear, open channel of communication, each employee has the

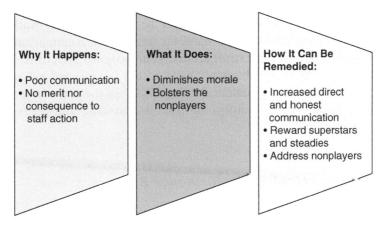

Why It Happens:

• Poor communication
• No merit nor consequence to staff action

What It Does:

• Diminishes morale
• Bolsters the nonplayers

How It Can Be Remedied:

• Increased direct and honest communication
• Reward superstars and steadies
• Address nonplayers

FIGURE 4–2.   Loss of trust.

opportunity to explore the parameters of his or her relationship with you. Apprehension can be addressed, questions can be answered, and directions can be ascertained through clear communication. Employees can gain a sense of their new leader's style through this mode of communication. Without it, the perception can arise that game playing or selective communication is the new manager's modus operandi.

Start building your communication strategy by remembering to ask questions frequently to all members of your staff. Utilize the questions provided in this book, and focus specifically on asking them what can be done to make the organization better and what they need from you in order to become better workers. The second approach is to ensure that monthly department meetings are held so that employees can discuss work progress and you can review your goals and objectives for the organization. The third strategy is to try to analyze which staff members need the most (or least) communication. Make an entry in your manager's logbook about how often you will meet with each individual on a one-to-one, interpersonal basis. This will give more reticent staff members an opportunity to discuss issues they might not feel comfortable addressing openly in a meeting.

Many managers advocate an open-door policy. This is a good idea in theory, but in practice it requires some fine-tuning. Establish certain hours during which your door is indeed open and workers can have access to you. Ask your assistant or secretary (if you have one) to screen employee requests for meetings with you and to schedule them based on priority of need.

In addition to an open-door policy, apply the **management-by-walking-around** techniques. This strategy mandates setting aside a certain amount of time each day to simply stroll around your assigned area of responsibility, make sure that individuals have access to you, and ask questions in a nonthreatening manner. Again, this keeps the communication lines open while visibly reinforcing trust and making you accessible to your employees.

Holding Performance Reviews

Another way to establish trust is to pursue opportunities to review the past. Discuss with your staff areas in which their past performance was good or inferior. Ask for their suggestions on how improvement might be made. This can be done within the context of group performance or individual performance.

Reviewing Group Performance

Encourage staff to be direct and candid about their assessment of past performance as a group. Keep the conversation focused on performance, not on personality-based issues. For example, discourage reference to your predecessor's personality, that of individuals within the department, or other potentially explosive issues. In emphasizing performance, you discover areas for improvement and crystallize specific methods on how to improve performance throughout the department and within individual work roles.

Discussion about "what we are doing wrong" also helps establish trust. By acknowledging that the department is not perfect and that you as a manager will not be perfect, you remind everyone involved that you share the human quality of imperfection. This listing of mistakes and opportunities for improvement is a good opener in establishing trust. Most healthcare workers are perfectionists who strive for ideal outcomes in all their assigned responsibilities. Accordingly, they are well versed not only on what goes wrong but why it went wrong. By reviewing mistakes and concentrating on where a problem might exist, your staff might understand your identity with them resonantly and therefore feel free to share their thoughts on areas for improvement.

To use this strategy in a practical application, have all members in your department or work group brainstorm areas for improvement.

Challenges	Controllables	Uncontrollables
– Training program for new employees on how ACOs work – Rollout of new benefit package	– Several members of the staff know how ACOs work – A new state grant can help provide training on the new benefit package	– No one is really sure how ACOs will impact the urban community of the hospital – Several employees are bound to **act up** and/or **act out** at the benefit info sessions

FIGURE 4–3.   Sample of change/crisis charting.

Using an easel (as a group) or individual notepads, they can divide the page into three columns. In the first column list is the event or application that needs improvement. For the second column, ask your staff to focus in on things they can control or are doing right relative to the problems/challenges cited in column 1. Also ask for suggestions for improvement as part of a commitment to the continuous quality improvement process to your work activities. In the third column, have them list situations and circumstances of which the department has either limited or no control.

Figure 4–3 shows an example of this charting system as used by a hospital's human resource department. The first column lists challenges; the second contains entries of things within their control; the third indicates problems with a project or process they feel are out of their control.

In later sessions (or regular department meetings), you might want to discuss as a group how the team can become stronger. This could include another exercise on how the team can meet the needs of the customer/patient at an even higher level of quality and effectiveness. Five basic questions can be used in this regard and can be added easily to the agenda of your monthly meeting. These questions are:

1. Where does communication seem to break down?
2. When do we operate as a team most efficiently?
3. When do we operate as a team least efficiently?

4. On a scale of 1 to 10, how would you rate the level of pride we have in our department (1 = very proud; 5 = no pride)?

5. What can we do better as a group?

As always, there is no **magic answer** to any one question. These questions serve to facilitate a group process for discussion of specific areas needing improvement and, more directly, to address areas in which the unit can work more strongly as a team; problems are defined and solutions are formed; (eg, patient parking could be a problem raised by the group, and rerouting of cars by members of the hospital security team could be the solution). This, along with other strategies in this book, can be a logical (and immediate) starting point from which to establish trust. It also sets a precedent for discussion of issues from a team perspective so those workers view themselves a group in which no one wins unless everyone wins.

Reviewing Individual Performance

The people rowing the boat do not have time to rock the boat. Translated, this means that if you can immediately establish trust on an individual employee basis, each worker will be vested with advancing the group process. Sit down as soon as possible with each employee to discuss privately his or her job, perceived role in the organization, and needs. You should do most of the listening while the staff member does most of the talking. Prepare several questions to help frame this one-on-one meeting; their purpose is to elicit a specific response, guide the discussion, and initiate what should become a healthy manager-staff relationship.

Some suggested questions for these individual meetings are:

• Tell me about your history here at [name of hospital].

• What do you need to become better at your job?

• How can I best support you in your everyday activities?

• What qualities do you look for in a supervisor?

• What short-term plans do you have in your job?

• What long-term plans do you have in your job?

• What are some of the major aspirations for your career?

• What advice do you have for me as I begin in my role as department manager?

These questions have used by many healthcare managers in our consulting work and have reaped great benefits in beginning a strong manager-employee dialogue and providing a sound starting point in the manager-staff member relationship.

Setting Policies and Standards

In establishing trust, it is important to set standards immediately in your work role. As discussed in other chapters, it is important to communicate to all department members your policies and standards. These could be communicated via memo, or better yet, individually and in group meetings. These policies should include a simple overview of your management style, your key expectations for the department, and what you expect from each member in terms of job performance.

In the interest of clarity and simplicity, the best approach is usually to say generally that you expect four things from each department member: **full effort, clear communication relative to individual needs and desires on the job, respect and dignity in the workplace, and compliance with all organization standards.** Using this as a building block, you can present more detailed direction and standards in the near future relative to technical items, work projects, and interpersonal dealings. As always, by your own words and actions as a leader—which will be closely observed by all members of your work group—your departmental standards will become fuller, clearer, and more integrated into daily workplace activities. If people know where they stand and all individual members are **rowing the boat, trust flourishes**.

Providing Clear Direction and Feedback

A system of clear direction and feedback is an imperative in the healthcare setting, where direction and timely feedback can spell the difference between good health and bad health and between life and death. Take every opportunity to instruct your employees, provide assistance, and give them the benefit of your technical acumen. This creates a sense of trust among employees, particularly when your input helps forward individual success. As always, asking intelligent questions is the hallmark of good leadership. Figure 4–4 provides a roster of very effective, field-proven questions which can be used in this regard. Not only does it convey interest in the employee's activities, it demonstrates that you are in a learning mode.

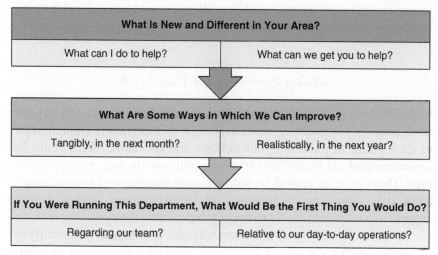

What Is New and Different in Your Area?	
What can I do to help?	What can we get you to help?

What Are Some Ways in Which We Can Improve?	
Tangibly, in the next month?	Realistically, in the next year?

If You Were Running This Department, What Would Be the First Thing You Would Do?	
Regarding our team?	Relative to our day-to-day operations?

FIGURE 4–4. Asking the right questions.

Downplaying Minutiae

Another route to establishing trust is to downplay minutiae, those trivialities that have little or no impact on overall departmental performance. However, use your judgment and exercise diplomacy—something that might seem trivial or inconsequential to you might be very important to an employee.

For example, in a major metropolitan hospital, conflict and a lack of trust became a problem because of the way groups of workers took their breaks on shift. Basically, a personality conflict arose because a new supervisor mistakenly made a big deal out of cliques going on break at the same time (which had been allowed by the previous supervisor). To remedy the situation and to underscore trust, the manager's new tactic was to state that he/she did not care who went on break with whom, just that everyone performed when it was time to perform. By stating this standard, as well as downplaying a small symptom that was really a sign of a bigger problem in the work situation, the manager refocused his/her staff's activities and performance emphasis, to the point where the issue of break time became immaterial.

Reevaluating Operations From Time to Time

A final tip on establishing trust is to reevaluate your work group from time to time. This is done using all the techniques cited in this section at various times throughout your initial year as a departmental manager. This includes having meetings, on both an individual and a group basis from time to time, to reexamine the questions discussed in this section. By revisiting these areas, you will ensure that trust is part of the continuum of performance and departmental activity. In establishing trust, you now have a basis on which individuals will promulgate pride throughout the work group and leave most of the conflict of the past exactly where it belongs—in the past. Finally, the avenues of communication will be open and will become part of the everyday process to act proactively to avoid future conflict among department members.

INTRADEPARTMENTAL CONFLICT AND RESOLUTION

Despite your best efforts to establish trust throughout the work group and to avoid potential conflict, human nature will unfortunately create occasions for intradepartmental conflict throughout your tenure as a healthcare manager. This unfortunate reality is defined as any conflict that takes place within your department or work group. This section will discuss the symptoms of intradepartmental conflict and present various solutions for resolving conflict so that progressive action and quality of performance become the department's top priority.

Symptoms of Intradepartmental Conflict

To begin with, intradepartmental conflict takes place on an interpersonal basis. That is why so many clichés for example—"**personality conflict**," "**not part of the team**," and "**tough to deal with**"—are used when describing conflict. Interpersonal conflict, particularly within a work group, is potentially the most damaging type of problem a healthcare manager can deal with, because it is implosive by nature; that is, it explodes from within. An atomic bomb, for example, explodes simply because the nucleus explodes first, which then creates adverse reaction throughout all layers of the atom. In a similar vein, when interpersonal conflict exists within a department, implosion can occur that, if not abated and healed, eventually can have drastic negative consequences for the entire department.

Numerous indicators signal intradepartmental conflict. These symptoms should be looked at using your own instincts and observation and examined in a cause-and-effect fashion. Following is a list of potential symptoms, their potential cause, and certainly their effect on your department. They are examined within the parameters of a departmental relationship.

Anger: Interpersonal adversity, loss of temper, lack of patience, or flat-out confrontational behavior can be exhibited in certain kinds of interpersonal conflict.

Avoidance: Avoidance occurs when an individual declines to work with someone and simply avoids contact with that person. The effect of this is that work may not be done and that establishment of team process may be compromised. Avoidance is more subtle than anger, which is direct in nature.

Blame: Individuals will often blame one another for mistakes or cite another individual as a reason for their own inability or failure to perform. Blaming creates hostility among team members and betrays basic trust and pride in the organization.

Excuse making: One individual will use another's behavior as an excuse for not performing a particular task. He or she may focus specifically on a personality nuance as being the problem that gets in the way of accomplishment. Another form of making excuses it to rationalize the negative behavior of others; for example, "Well you can't expect too much from so-and-so, you know how they are"; this form of excusing relies on a personality trait as the reason for nonperformance or inadequate performance.

Isolation and fragmentation: Over time, certain team members may exclude one or more players due to personality conflict. The effect of isolation is that participation in the group process is jeopardized. Ultimately, there is a withdrawal of the resources needed to get the job done. Exclusion can occur to the point that workers may become isolated from the organization or organize their own faction. This fragmentation can become particularly deleterious in any group process, especially those that require emergency response.

Confrontation: Certain personality types are argumentative by nature, so that even routine operations are interrupted by confrontation and overall disruption of group harmony. This is a waste of time as well as a demoralizer.

Criticism: Over the long term, an individual who is critical of everything and everyone in the department also creates a morale problem.

Ironically, others respond to this behavior by becoming defensive and in turn critical of the chronic criticizer.

Erosion of performance levels: Ill feeling, over time, leads to diminished performance among workers. Some begin to look for another workplace if the situation is not corrected by the manager.

Regression: Continued erosion of performance leads to regression. In an era where health care must be progressive, every employee's performance must contribute to its maximum potential.

Resolving Intradepartmental Conflict

To resolve intradepartmental conflict, an assortment of solutions can be employed. What they have in common, however, is a need to identify the symptoms, recognize the full effects of the conflict, and work through the issues with staff so that resolution can be arrived at with confidence.

Identifying Symptoms

To begin with, identify the symptoms of conflict, using as a basis the list in the preceding section. Look for the source of conflicts, specifically who is creating it and what the root cause may be. Note behavior or language that may provoke problems. This could include derogatory terms used to describe certain team members; the **silent treatment** directed toward particular team members; or outright verbal conflict or nonverbal hostility, such as glaring and gestures of disapproval.

Recognizing Effects of Conflict

Recognize what effect the situation may have on the entire group. First try to define whether the conflict is an individual versus a group problem; an individual versus individual problem; or a group versus a group (faction) problem. This will help you to be more specific not only in symptom identification, but also in a potential solution.

Try to quantify the person's (or group) behavior as much as possible by recording in your logbook as many specific incidents as you can. Then use your notes to analyze whether the problem is related to poor attitude, lack of interpersonal skills, team orientation, or technical ability. To educate the employee(s) and to correct the problem later, you must be as specific as possible and collect as many examples as feasible. This evidence will help you illustrate the problem to the employee or group and to provide the education needed to correct it.

Next, determine the full extent of an interpersonal problem—primarily whether it is limited to or whether it is having a contagious effect on others in the department who were not initially involved. Try to ascertain whether a faction is being created by the problem or if one individual seems to be deliberately gathering support from others to form a faction. It is essential to stop the spread of harmful intradepartmental conflict as early as possible.

Working Through Issues

After collecting and analyzing your information, approach the responsible party (parties) directly. In general, five steps should be taken to resolve intradepartmental conflict: separate into two distinct categories for fluid discussion and reach agreement on their relative importance, discuss harmful performance and its effects, explore the causes of conflict, state your expectations for resolution, and express confidence in arriving at a solution. Setting parameters for both staff participation (Figure 4–5) and house rules for conduct (Figure 4–6) is essential to both this effort and the maintenance of morale and trust in your department, and among your team.

Separate the issues into two categories. First identify the business-related attributes of the problem-business outcomes, performance dimensions, and technical areas. Then list personal issues that might bear on the conflict. These include any of the 10 symptoms set forth earlier—anger, avoidance, blame, and so forth—as well as your own observations from your logbook.

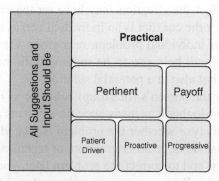

FIGURE 4–5.   Parameters for participation.

• Appropriate humor and laughing only • No gossip, politics, or polemics onstage • Every problem posed must have a suggested solution • Anytime is a good time to get help as needed	• It's us, not they • Keep personal conversations backstage and away from patients • We do **everything** here; no patient need cannot be met

FIGURE 4–6. House rules.

Review this information completely with the involved party and reach consensus on the facts of the issues. If no one acknowledges the facts, you might have to state more directly your belief in their validity and supplement that statement with the pledge that you will not accept this behavior any further.

Next, move the discussion to performance, focusing specifically on the business effects from the conflict. Cite work that is not being done; explain what effect the employee's (or group's) behavior has on other department members, and how this behavior interferes with others getting their jobs done. Discuss further how this behavior affects other departments and, most important, the customers/patients. By all means, use your own technical acumen to explain the specific negative consequence of the behavior and the danger if it continues.

Third, ask why this behavior has taken place and how it might be corrected. Try to get to the bottom of what they believe is contributing to the problem and how the cause might be alleviated. Following this discussion, present your own ideas on why the problem exists; however, spend most of your discussion on how the problem must be remedied.

Fourth, state clearly, concisely, and resolutely your expectations, standards, and policies for future action. Explain what will be accepted by you as satisfactory behavior and, moreover, what will be considered poor performance or interpersonal conflict. These include probation or any other disciplinary action, including termination.

Finally, express your confidence that the situation will be corrected and ask if particular assistance is needed to do so. Try to strike a delicate balance between expressing optimism that the situation can be corrected and underscoring the fact that continued poor performance and intradepartmental conflict will not be tolerated under any conditions.

As you deal with the difficult task of resolving intradepartmental conflict, you should incorporate two strategies into your efforts. The first is to do a precise, effective, and efficient job of fact-finding every step of the way, as detailed in the section on "Resolving Intradepartmental Conflict." The second strategy for resolving intradepartmental conflict is through policy compliance. Utilize as needed your facility's personnel policies and its expertise to resolve the problem. Also, rely on your own manager's input. In some cases, you might want someone from the human resource department or your manager to sit in with you as you seek resolution with the conflicted parties. This not only gives you some assistance and support, it also conveys to those involved in the conflict that this is a serious matter that will be dealt with resolutely. This does not demonstrate any weakness on your part. In fact, it shows strength because it indicates to the employee that you have the clout with which to resolve the problem. To further get this message across, take the lead in the conversation and state your expectations for the department as well as promising further discipline if the problem is not corrected.

To gain the most benefit from your personnel policies, use both your documentation notebook to record counseling sessions and the performance evaluation. Clear documentation notes and subsequent notation on the performance evaluation will once again stress the importance to the employee or group that intradepartmental conflict is not an accepted mode of behavior on the job. Whichever approach you take, make sure that all involved parties understand clearly the consequences if performance and conflict are not remedied.

Interpersonal conflict, particularly within a department, is complex and can hinder progressive action. Again, it must be dealt with in a timely fashion, resolutely, and with a certain force of character so that the majority of your department is not adversely affected. Remember, an array of individuals look to you for leadership. By not dealing ethically and promptly with interpersonal conflict, you not only encourage substandard performance, you also abdicate the trust and leadership your organization and staff expect from you. If the suggestions in this section are followed, this difficult area of management can become less burdensome and more productive.

TERMINATION AND PROBATION

Knowing **when** to fire someone is as difficult as knowing **how** to do it. In the words of a healthcare manager at a client facility in the Southwest, "When I fire someone, I'm also firing their family." This underscores the difficulty attached to terminating an employee. However, terminating employees is an unfortunate but necessary part of being a healthcare manager. When individual performance has deteriorated to the point of being counterproductive, it is clearly time for separation. In many cases, individuals are actually relieved when terminated, because they have become frustrated and ineffective in their work role.

Do not expect anyone to thank you for terminating them, however, or to admit that it was their fault for being terminated. Terminating an employee is a very difficult undertaking, and this section will review a 10-point checklist for signs that indicate that termination may need to be considered. How to make the termination process as painless and productive as possible will also be discussed.

Disciplinary probation is generally acknowledged as being a 3-month process in which a poor performer is given the opportunity, usually as **one last chance**, to make good on his or her employment obligation. Simply put, the individual has 3 months to turn performance around to an acceptable level. Most healthcare managers think that probation is a farce because if an individual **behaves** for 3 months, there is no guarantee that he or she will perform steadily for the rest of the year. In fact, they believe performance will usually regress. Probation is seen as a final step before termination and thus will get little discussion in this section.

Discuss with your personnel department the probation policy at your organization, for example, when an individual should go on probation. In many cases, an employee who is on probation will **terminate** himself or herself by securing other employment while on probation, thus saving you the headache of having to fire them. In this regard, probation is a worthwhile practice and should be used in conjunction with a performance evaluation for an employee who will be terminated eventually anyway. Beyond being used as a prelude to termination, probation has very little effect on performance enhancement. However, several guidelines can be used to help you decide whether to terminate an employee and if so, when and how.

When to Terminate

When should you fire someone? This question is asked during each of more than 50 seminars the authors conduct each year for healthcare managers and executives. The answer is not simple, as each case deals with a unique individual and specific circumstances. You should terminate an employee if more than seven of the following conditions prevail:

1. **Chronic poor attitude:** An employee who regularly appears to be inflexible, overly aggressive or confrontational, irresolute, tunnel-visioned, and displays a poor work ethic and no sense of industry, termination is indicated. Rarely are individuals who demonstrate these attitudes likely to change, because such outlooks are elemental to their personality and are life conditioning. In an industry that requires high adaptability, appropriately assertive behavior, perseverance, and a strong work ethic, these problems, which probably cannot be corrected, are unacceptable.

2. **Poor interpersonal skills:** An individual who consistently demonstrates interpersonal behavior problems and creates conflicts, as discussed earlier in the chapter, might be a candidate for termination. In a people-oriented field such as health care, poor interpersonal skill do not make for long-term success.

3. **Negative effect on others:** When an employee's negative behavior creates intradepartmental conflict and the employee has been counseled several times about the effect caused by these conflicts, termination must be considered.

4. **Poor performance documentation:** If the employee's pattern of performance documentation over a 1-year period has been largely negative, termination must be considered. Such an individual not only will fail to grow and develop on the job, he or she will actually regress to a level of performance that is less than what was expected this year. In short, an individual who has demonstrated a full year of poor performance has probably fallen into a pattern that will not be remedied by probation or another year on the job. In essence, he or she is absorbing a salary that can be better spent on a better performer.

5. **Gut instincts:** If you sense that it is time for the person to go, based on the first four factors cited in this section, termination probably is in order. Do not try to rationalize or over intellectualize your feelings.

6. **Counseling:** After a problem employee has been counseled by you, the human resource department, or other appropriate individuals in your organization, and still fails to perform acceptably, chances are the situation is not resolvable.

7. **Outside negative input:** If a customer/patient, peer, colleagues, or other department members have constructively criticized the individual's performance, most likely the performance is affecting the entire work flow of your department. To keep this problem from festering, termination must be enacted.

8. **Detrimental effect on organization:** A poor performer who is in a critical work position can adversely affect the entire organization. If you have clear evidence that this is the case, termination must be enacted quickly in order to keep organization integrity and strong performance at a premium.

9. **Regressive patterns, trends, and habits:** A person who consistently demonstrates poor on-the-job behavior, inappropriate work personality, and poor work habits—all substantiated by your own documentation—is a candidate for termination.

10. **Poor future outlook:** Ask the question, "Do you think the person will really turn it around?" If the answer is no, make your move.

Figure 4–7 contains a targeted checklist of additional indicators that can be used to help you evaluate whether you need to terminate an employee.

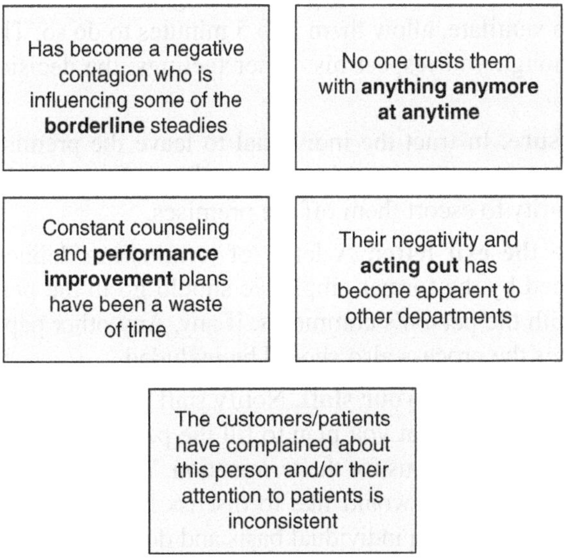

Has become a negative contagion who is influencing some of the **borderline** steadies	No one trusts them with **anything anymore at anytime**
Constant counseling and **performance improvement** plans have been a waste of time	Their negativity and **acting out** has become apparent to other departments

The customers/patients have complained about this person and/or their attention to patients is inconsistent

FIGURE 4–7.   Termination checkpoints.

How to Terminate

Having determined that termination is necessary, you now need to learn how to accomplish the task. Again, a 10-point checklist should help you through what is, at best, a difficult process.

1. **Explain documentation.** All prior appropriate documentation should be on hand for presentation at the time of termination. Explain in 2 to 3 minutes your overriding documentation and the reasons you considered termination as the only possible remedy. Documentation must be used as the basis for any discussion of termination.

2. **Recap performance counseling.** Quickly summarize all efforts made to resolve the performance problem.

3. **Get to the point.** Once steps 1 and 2 have been done, get to the point. Tell the individual that you are terminating them for cause. If the employee already guessed that he or she is being terminated and says so, simply acknowledge it and move on to the next step.

4. **Have a witness on hand.** If you have never fired an employee, ask that a third person (your boss or someone from the human resource department) be present at the session. This allows you to have support on hand as well as someone to help guide you through the process.

5. **Allow a monologue.** If the person being fired feels like talking or wants to ventilate, allow them 3 to 5 minutes to do so. Then respond that although you respect his or her feelings, the decision has been made.

6. **Get closure.** Instruct the individual to leave the premises, but first explain the procedure for cleaning out his or her desk. If necessary, call security to escort them off the premises.

7. **Prepare the exit letter.** A letter of termination delineating cause and signed by the former employee should go in the personnel file, along with the person's comments, if any. Any other paperwork that completes the process also should be included.

8. **Communicate with your staff.** Notify staff that you have terminated the individual and that you plan to fill the position quickly. You need not disclose the reasons for the termination. Tell them that it was your decision, but if they would like to discuss it further, they can come into your office on an individual basis and do so. If further discussion is desired, only the future of the department should be discussed, not the terminated employee (eg, "Now we will have to...")

9. **Reject additional input.** Once an employee has been terminated, you need not accept further **input** from another employee. Your focus should be on the future, specifically on employee suggestions for filling the position. This keeps the termination on a professional basis.

10. **Fill the position quickly.** Quickly filling the position of a terminated employee is the best remedy for this situation. You have an opportunity to command trust and allegiance from your staff by providing them with a productive, professional new colleague.

Termination is never easy, but by utilizing these techniques and enlisting the support of your superiors and human resource staff, you can move through this difficult situation.

DEALING WITH INTERNAL AND EXTERNAL CUSTOMERS

A final tough situation you will need to manage in dealing with the complaints of internal customers (such as physicians and unions) and external customers (such as patients and customer-payers).

External Customers

In dealing with customer/patient complaints, again it is important to first do your fact-finding. Resources include the customer/patient and any staff members who might have dealt with the customer/patient. Ask questions and listen carefully to all information provided and take notes for accuracy and to show empathy for what is being said. These notes can also act as a chronology in resolving the problem. Move proactively and try to head off future complaints by handling this one as quickly as possible. Use your perception to get a full picture of the situation and the basis for the complainant's anger or dissatisfaction. By all means, accept responsibility for any disservice and promise the customer/patient that definitive follow-up action will take place and feedback will be provided.

Remembering that most customers/patients fall into 3 categories of behavior, as indicated in Figure 1–4, is important in these efforts and can help you in strategy formulation.

As part of the investigation stage, ask those who worked with the customer/patient their version of what happened. Use your facility's chain of command to get support whenever possible. Then resolve the situation by calling the customer/patient directly, explaining the problem, and writing a follow-up letter of empathy. Offer to provide any corrective action as appropriate, making certain to document the entire episode and refer action to appropriate sources. As always with interpersonal interaction, communication is critical. Always remember that unlike a retail situation where another product or a coupon can be given to a customer, customers/patients in the healthcare setting require empathy and the promise that a harmful action will not take place again. Very serious actions or requests from the customer/patient should be referred to the appropriate source, usually your supervisor.

Internal Customers

In the case of internal customers—notably, physicians and union members—other strategies for handling complaints should be used. For physicians, there are 6 keys to sound physician relations:

1. A strong organization orientation to meeting the legitimate needs of physicians in serving their patients
2. Inclusion of physicians in departmental activities and events
3. Consistent communication
4. Professional support
5. Shared views on meeting the needs of customers/patients
6. Cohesive efforts to ensure an effective and efficient flow of work

First and foremost, physicians should always be part of the team and be included in as many activities and meetings as possible. Many healthcare organizations have physicians contribute to newsletters or involve them in strategic planning and hiring decisions.

Whenever possible, ask physicians for advice on how you can better support their responsibilities. Discuss every physician's complaint with the medical director and physician in a three-way meeting. Again, utilize the questions appearing in the Practical Resource section as part of your practicum, acting as quickly as possible and using all available communications channels. Many newly appointed healthcare managers create problems for themselves by starting off **on the wrong foot** with physicians.

Get to know the medical staff, as well as all members of your organization, so that you will have access to all available resources when resolving internal customer complaints.

A final source of potential conflict within your organization's customer base is the union employee. With union drives being an ongoing presence in healthcare organizations, it is important to maintain your managerial equilibrium at all times and remain neutral during union elections and other labor relations' activity. Answer all questions objectively; do not try to win over votes from individuals who are prounion or those who are decidedly antiunion. Rather, try to provide support for individuals who are undecided and thus pressured by both sides. Reassure employees that life will go on despite the outcome of a union election, and stay close to your human resource department to keep up with developments and learn essential information you might need. Remember, union activity is no excuse for poor performance; therefore, continue to note poor performance in your logbook throughout union activity.

When dealing with all customer complaints, remember to show compassion, take command, and communicate with all responsible parties. The best way to enhance your credibility in conflict situation is to seek answers, decide on action, and execute that action resolutely.

SUMMARY

In all conflict situations, do what is most compatible with your management style. Given that conflict is not a comfortable situation, and managing tough situations is not the most appealing part of your management agenda, trust your gut instincts and trust your power of observation. By being concerned about the welfare of your entire staff as well as your customers/patients and colleagues throughout the organization, you will demonstrate a consistency that will help establish your credibility as a manager.

Keep in mind the following five factors of mediating conflict and managing tough situations: **compassion, concern, communication, comfort, and command.** These will help establish your managerial credibility, which is so vital to establishing trust and the personal power base you will need to manage tough situations effectively. Once you have used some of the techniques discussed in this chapter and established your own comfort zone with these strategies, these tough situations will be more manageable and your overall management systems more effective.

PRACTICAL RESOURCE—CHAPTER IV:
Change Strategy Guide

OVERVIEW

Change is a constant in health care, as we have discussed through our text. This guide will help you proactively and progressively plan for change and garner maximum participation and positive action from your staff.

CHANGE STRATEGY GUIDE

This worksheet is essentially a simple brainstorming tool that can be utilized individually or collectively and helps to discern a realistic plan of action during times of change.

> **Need(s) for change—apparent**
> -
> -
> -

> **Need(s) for change—not clearly evident**
> -
> -
> -

> **Major objective(s) of the change**
> -
> -
> -

> **Primary benefits**
> -
> -
> -

> **Secondary benefits**
> -
> -
> -

Major fears of staff members, in general

-

-

-

Major fears of staff members, credible

-

-

-

Major fears of staff members, nonplayer driven

-

-

-

Significant obstacles

-

-

-

Potential solutions to obstacles

-

-

-

-

-

Prevailing related perceptions—positive

-

-

-

-

Prevailing related perceptions—negative

-

-

-

-

Indicators of success (percentages, time measurements, money/finance signs, and significant tracking numbers)

-
-
-
-
-

Potential milestone/critical junctures of change process

-
-
-
-
-

LEADERSHIP KEYS FOR SIGNIFICANT PLAYERS IN THE CHANGE

Direct reports and technical experts

-
-
-
-

Superstars/action agents

-
-
-
-

Steadies/advocates

-
-
-
-

Nonplayers

-
-
-
-

Resource needs (cash, personnel, equipment, technical support, and leadership guidance)

-
-
-
-

Time/event chart of major action—4 significant junctures

-
-
-
-

MAJOR 5 COMMUNICATION MESSAGES ABOUT THIS CHANGE

-
-
-
-
-

Major benefits of the change to

Customer/patient

-
-
-

Organization

-
-
-

Team

-

-

-

Individual staff member

-

-

-

CHAPTER FIVE

Practical Strategy for Planning

THE ESSENTIAL ELEMENTS OF SUCCESSFUL PLANS

All successful plans have four major features:

- Organize processes, procedures, and staff for efficient and effective work.
- Influence and lead team members or employees who report to you.
- Monitor work progress, schedules, and budgets.
- Identify problems and suggest corrective actions.

The following section explores the importance of planning, the basic types of plans healthcare managers work with, the step-by-step way plans are created, and a host of special tools and techniques that can make plans more effective and efficient for everyone who utilizes them.

In today's demanding healthcare workplace, your department, team, or workgroup needs to consistently meet goals both large and small to help improve the overall company as well as your specific group. Meeting—and, hopefully, exceeding these goals and expectations—enables your department and company to become ever better at what they do, staying one step ahead of the competition. Healthcare organizations face pressures and challenges from many sources, all of which increase the importance of good planning. External forces include competition, increased government regulations, ever-more complex technologies, the uncertainties of a global economy, and rising labor and resource costs. Internal forces include the demand for greater efficiency, increased diversity in the workforce, and the introduction of new processes, structures, and work arrangements.

In today's ever-changing work environment, good planning offers a number of benefits and advantages for your employees, your teammates, and even your own career.

GREATER FOCUS AND FLEXIBILITY

Good planning improves focus and flexibility for both you and your organization.

- **Focus:** An organization with focus knows what it does best, knows the needs of its customers or patients, and knows how to serve them well. An individual with focus knows where he or she wants to go in a career or situation and is able to keep that objective in mind, even in difficult circumstances.

- **Flexibility:** An organization with flexibility is willing and able to change and adapt to shifting circumstances and operates by looking toward the future (rather than the past or present). An individual with flexibility balances his or her career plans with the problems and opportunities posed by new and developing circumstances—both personal and organizational.

THE PLANNING PROCESS

At its most basic, planning is decision making. When you plan, you use information to make plans that address significant problems and opportunities. Figure 5–1 shows a typical approach to decision making as applied during the **planning process**. The planning process begins with identification of a problem and ends with evaluation of implemented solutions. This section covers each step of the planning process in detail, addressing the key responsibilities of managers at each phase.

There are 5 steps in the planning process:

Step 1: Identify and define the problem.

Step 2: Generate and evaluate possible courses of action.

Step 3: Choose a preferred solution.

Step 4: Implement the solution.

Step 5: Evaluate results.

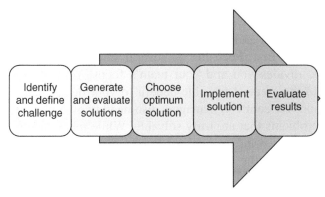

FIGURE 5-1. The 5 stages of planning.

Identify and Define the Problem

During the first step of planning and decision making—finding and defining the problem—you gather information, evaluate information, and deliberate. Problem symptoms usually signal the presence of a performance deficiency or opportunity.

During this step, you need to assess the situation properly by looking beyond symptoms to find out what is really happening. Take special care to not just address a symptom while ignoring the true problem. The way you define a problem originally can have a major impact on how you go about resolving it. Poor problem definition can lead to poor or ineffective plans, and the following three common mistakes:

- **Focusing on symptoms instead of causes.** Symptoms indicate that problems may exist, but don't mistake them for the problems themselves. Most managers can spot problem symptoms (like a drop in an employee's performance). Instead of treating symptoms (such as simply encouraging higher performance), good managers need to address the symptom's root causes (in this case, discovering that the worker's need for additional training in how to use a complex new computer system).

- **Defining the problem too broadly or too narrowly.** To take a classic example, the problem stated as **build a better mousetrap** can be more broadly defined as **get rid of the mice now**. That is, managers should define problems so as to give themselves the best possible range of planning options.

- **Choosing the wrong problem to deal with.** Managers need to set priorities and make plans that deal with the most important problems first. Focusing on several small, less-important initiatives divides you and your team's focus. Your efforts may not yield the greatest possible benefit to your department or organization. By contrast, managers also need to give planning priority to problems that are truly solvable. While many healthcare managers may want to overhaul the Medicare system, focusing on streamlining the Medicare billing processes for your department is a much more achievable goal for you and your teammates.

A variety of tools and techniques help managers identify and define problems, as we will see in a later section of this chapter.

Generate and Evaluate Possible Courses of Action

After you define the problem, you can begin formulating one or several potential solutions. At this stage of planning and decision making, you may need to gather more information, evaluate data, analyze internally and externally gathered statistics, and weigh the pros and cons of each possible course of action. Involving others during this planning stage is critical in order to develop a range of solutions, get the most out of available information, and build future commitment for the plan.

Your plan will only be as good as the quality of the alternative solutions you generate during this step. The better the pool of alternatives, the more likely a good solution can be achieved. A very basic evaluation used at this step is

- Cost-benefit analysis, which compares alternative costs (time, money, resources, human capital, etc) to the expected benefits. At a minimum, the benefits of a preferred alternative should be greater than its costs. Although cost-benefit analysis is often quantitative (based on measurable facts and figures), the results need to be tempered by your subjective, qualitative judgments to ensure full evaluation of the options.

Choose a Preferred Course of Action

At this stage in the planning process, you must make a decision and select a particular course of action. Exactly how you make a decision and who may need to weigh in on the decision varies for each planning situation. In some cases, you may determine the best alternative by using cost-benefit analysis criterion; share this choice with your manager, and then proceed with executing your plan. Other times, numerous criteria may come into play, and you may need to present the case for your decision to multiple committees and managers, gradually getting others to buy into your solution. However, after you generate and evaluate the alternatives, you must make a final choice to continue in the planning process.

You should test any decision to follow a particular plan of action by performing an ethics check. This evaluation ensures that you properly consider the ethical aspects of working in today's complex, fast-changing work environment.

Implement the Planned Course of Action

After you select the preferred solution to a problem, you next establish and implement appropriate actions to meet your final goal. This is the stage at which you finally set directions and initiate problem-solving actions.

Nothing new can happen according to the plan unless action is taken. Managers not only need the determination and creativity to make a plan, but they also need the ability and willingness to implement it. Additionally, most successful plans require managers and others to take some sort of action. Many plans fail at this stage because a manager didn't adequately involve others and gain their support. Managers who use participation wisely get the right people involved in decisions and problem solving from the beginning. When they do, plans are more likely to be implemented quickly, smoothly, and to everyone's satisfaction.

Evaluate Results

Planning and decision making are not complete until you evaluate the results. In this final stage, you compare your accomplishments with your original objectives. If the desired results are not achieved, the process must be reviewed and renewed to allow for corrective actions. Remember to examine both the positive and negative consequences of a chosen course of action. If the original solution appears inadequate, a return to earlier steps may be required to generate a modified or new plan. Evaluation is also made easier if the original plan includes objectives with measurable targets and timetables.

PLANNING TOOLS AND TECHNIQUES

Planning is challenging in any circumstances, and the difficulties increase as the work environment becomes more uncertain. To help master these challenges, managers make use of a number of useful planning tools and techniques during the planning process and after a plan is put into place. Some of the most common planning tools and techniques include

- Forecasting
- Contingency planning
- Scenario planning
- Benchmarking
- Participation
- Strategic planning

Forecasting

Forecasting is the process of making assumptions about what will happen in the future. A forecast is a specific vision of the future. All good plans involve forecasts, particularly during Steps 1 and 2 of the planning process. Some forecasts are qualitative and use expert opinions to predict the future. In this case, a single person of special expertise or reputation or a panel of experts may be consulted. Other forecasts are quantitative and use mathematical and statistical analysis of data to predict future events.

In the final analysis, forecasting always relies on human judgment. Even the results of highly sophisticated quantitative forecasting still require interpretation and are subject to error. Forecasting is not planning—it is a planning tool. Treat forecasts cautiously, reviewing all information with a critical and questioning eye.

Contingency Planning

Planning always involves thinking ahead. But the more unstructured the problems and more uncertain the planning environment, the more likely that your original assumptions, predictions, and intentions may prove to be in error. Even the most carefully prepared plans may prove inadequate as experience develops. Unexpected problems and events frequently occur. When they do, plans have to be changed.

As a manager, you are better off anticipating problems than being surprised by them. **Contingency planning** is the process of identifying alternative courses of action that you can implement if and when an original plan proves inadequate because of changing circumstances. Sometimes contingency plans are created by good forward thinking on the part of managers and staff. At other times, a devil's advocate method, in which you formally assume the worst-case forecasts of future events and brainstorm responses, can yield effective contingency plans. Whatever methods you use to establish contingency plans, remember that the earlier the need for changes can be detected, the better. Look for **trigger points** in regular processes and procedures that can indicate that your existing plan is no longer desirable and needs to be closely monitored.

Scenario Planning

Scenario planning is a popular and long-term version of contingency planning. Scenario planning involves identifying several alternative future states of affairs that may occur. Managers and staff then deal hypothetically with each situation and formulate possible plans.

The creative brainstorming process helps organizations operate more flexibly in dynamic environments. The United States Marine Corps has been doing scenario planning for many years and in fact makes it a requisite of its leadership training. The process began years ago when instructors presented officer candidates with perplexing questions based on scenarios replicating crisis and combat situations. In a healthcare setting, similar questions can be posed by creating alternative future scenarios while remaining sensitive to the nature of growing environmental changes. Although recognizing that planning scenarios can never be inclusive of all future possibilities, these scenarios help **condition the organization to think** and remain better prepared than its competitors for **future shocks**.

Benchmarking

Another important influence on the success or failure of planning is the frame of reference used as a starting point. All too often, managers and planners have limited awareness of what is happening outside their immediate work setting. Successful planning must challenge the status quo; it cannot simply accept things the way they are.

Benchmarking is a technique that uses external comparisons to evaluate one's current performance and identify possible future actions; it is one tool that broadens a work group and organization's field of view. The purpose of benchmarking is to find out what other people and organizations are doing very well and plan how to incorporate these ideas into your own operations. Healthcare–specific benchmarking programs and Web sites—such as www.healthdatacheck.com—have emerged as useful tools to help healthcare managers track and compare performance.

Participation and Group Involvement

Participation is critical to the planning process. **Participative planning** involves the people who are affected by a plan or who are required to help implement the plan to aid in the planning process. Participation can increase the creativity and information available for planning. It can also increase the understanding, acceptance, and commitment of people to final plans. Indeed, planning in organizations should rarely, if ever, be done by individuals. To create and implement the best plans, others must be genuinely involved during all planning steps. Even though participative planning takes more time, it can improve results by improving implementation.

Strategic Planning

A **strategy** is a comprehensive action plan that identifies long-term direction and guides managers and staff in ways to best utilize the organization's resources. Successful strategic plans using resources focus an entire organization's energies on a clear target or goal. Usually strategic plans originate in the uppermost management and executive levels of a company. Smaller, more specific plans in departments, teams, or work groups need to mesh with and build on the overarching strategic plans.

Missions, Values, and Objectives

Mission statements, core values statements, and **objectives** are all strategic planning tools that help managers create plans that fit the organization's vision for the future of its business endeavors.

- **Mission:** An organization's reason for existence as a supplier of goods and/or services to society. A good mission statement is precise in identifying where the organization intends to operate, who the organization serves, and what products or services it provides. The best organizations have clear and compelling missions. At the Breast Cancer Program of the Dana-Farber-Harvard Cancer Center, the mission is "to reduce death due to breast cancer and lengthen and improve the quality of life of women with this disease." At Merck it is "to preserve and improve human life."

- **Core values:** Affect and guide the action of an organization. Often posted along with the organization's mission statement, these values reflect the organization's broad beliefs about what is and is not appropriate. The presence of strong core values gives character to an organization, backs up the mission statement, and helps guide the behavior of members in meaningful and consistent ways. For example, core values at Merck include corporate social responsibility, science-based innovation, honesty and integrity, and profit from work that benefits humanity.

- **Objectives:** Direct activities toward key and specific results. Whereas a mission statement sets forth an official purpose for the organization, objectives are usually shorter-term targets against which actual performance can be measured. Examples of business objectives may include producing at a certain level of profit, gaining and holding a specific share of a market, recruiting and maintaining a high-quality workforce, or making a positive contribution to society.

SWOT ANALYSIS

In order to produce effective plans, managers and staff must have a clear picture of what's happening within an organization and within its greater business environment. SWOT analysis (strengths, weaknesses, opportunities, and threats) is a common tool used to analyze strengths and weaknesses inside the organization and opportunities and threats outside the organization.

Internal Factors

A **SWOT analysis** begins with a systematic evaluation of an organization's resources and capabilities. A major goal is to identify **core competencies** in the form of special strengths that the organization has or does exceptionally well in comparison with competitors. Simply put, organizations need core competencies that do important things better than the competition and that are very difficult for competitors to duplicate. Core competencies may be found in special knowledge or expertise, outstanding technologies, unique products, or superior distribution systems, among many other possibilities.

- **Strengths:** The resources and capabilities an organization can use to develop competitive advantage
- **Weaknesses:** The absence of strengths

A major strategic goal of any organization is to create processes that highlight core competencies for competitive advantage by building upon organizational strengths and minimizing the impact of weaknesses.

External Factors

A SWOT analysis is not complete until opportunities and threats in the external environment are also analyzed.

- **Opportunities:** Include possible new markets, a strong economy, weaknesses in competitors, and emerging technologies
- **Threats:** Include the emergence of new competitors, scarce resources, changing customer demands, and new government regulations, among other possibilities

For the purpose of a SWOT analysis, the external environment includes macroenvironment factors such as technology, government, social structures, population demographics, the global economy, and the natural environment. The external environment also encompasses developments in the industry or business environment, which includes resource suppliers, competitors, customers, and patients.

In a stable and predictable external environment, you can more successfully implement a strategy for a longer period of time. By contrast, in a more dynamic and uncertain environment, you must choose flexible strategies that can change and evolve over time. Given the nature of competitive environments today, strategic management must be considered an ongoing process in which strategies are formulated, implemented, revised, and implemented again in a nearly continuous manner.

WHAT IT TAKES TO MAKE DECISIONS

Managerial decisions have direct impact on the work life and overall performance of other individuals. Given the limited resources in today's healthcare arena, managers also often make decisions that concern a number of areas: human resources, operational equipment, and financial expenditures, to name a few.

Every decision you make has consequence, not only on the work life of others, but also on the long-term progress of your department or team. As it seemed when you were a new physician and had to make decisions about the health of a patient, this responsibility may seem overwhelming; it is something managers must confront on a daily basis. Team members look to managers to direct their work activity, and the organization depends on managerial decisions to help effect positive action. Additionally, patients rely on managerial decisions for positive outcome with the health care they receive. This is especially pertinent when they are aware of the fact that the leader making the decision is a physician—someone who is perceived to be the most qualified and expert person in the entire continuum of their care.

Five essential values drive the decision-making process for managers:

- **Accountability:** Managers must use all the tools available to them in accomplishing their set goals. In addition, they must be accountable for how those resources are used. In analyzing data and taking into account the potential ramifications of their decisions, managers assume accountability on several levels. They must be accountable not only for the decision made, but also for how the decision was determined, what data were analyzed, and which course of action was pursued in arriving at the final decision.

- **Adaptability:** To demonstrate the flexibility needed for managing healthcare delivery in a turbulent business climate, managers must embrace a certain degree of adaptability. Adaptability means being flexible in considering options, being able to deal with a wide range of people, and having a versatile business approach. Managers must take care, however, to avoid being too adaptable; that is, becoming wishy-washy or irresolute by constantly straying from an established course of action, or spending so much time considering options that the manager ultimately fails to arrive at a set course of action.

- **Dependability:** Staff depends on leaders to make timely decisions that, for the most part, are correct and specify a proper course of action. Constant reluctance to take stands or making decisions without communication or staff input does not promote the perception among staff and the organization that a manager is dependable.

- **Responsibility:** A strong manager embraces responsibility for making decisions, takes ownership for decisions, and views the management role as a commitment to organizational excellence. These attitudes mandate selfless participation in the decision-making process so as to consider at all times what is good for the organization and to consider both the positive and negative ramifications of a decision on staff and the entire organization. (All decision making must be done while keeping in mind the organization's objective of providing stellar healthcare service to all its patients.) Managers who shirk responsibility may be seen as being overly political, figureheads, or worse. Even when managers delegate a particular task, they ultimately must take responsibility for the outcome.

- **Visibility:** Visible leaders are present and on the scene. In conducting their activities, they are around to hear the cheers and boos. Furthermore, a manager's visibility does not diminish in critical times or in situations that are out of the norm. At no time should a visible manager hear the question, "Who's in charge?"

UTILIZING THE PORTFOLIO PLANNING APPROACH

The **portfolio planning approach** is a basic method of formulating strategy and making decisions, in which managers allocate scarce organizational resources among competing opportunities. In the portfolio planning approach, resources include various products, services, business units, and departments or divisions.

This strategy employs an analysis of business opportunities according to market growth rate and market share. The matrix shows the following four possibilities, with each linked to a possible strategic direction.

- **Stars** are high-market-share opportunities in high-growth markets. They produce large profits through substantial penetration of expanding markets. The preferred strategy for stars is growth, and further resource investments in them are recommended.

- **Question marks** are low-market-share businesses in high-growth markets. They do not produce much profit but compete in rapidly growing markets. They are the source of difficult strategic decisions. The preferred strategy is growth, but the risk exists that further investments may not result in improved market share. The most promising question marks should be targeted for growth; others are retrenchment candidates.

- **Cash cows** are high-market-share businesses in low-growth markets. They produce large profits and a strong cash flow. Because the markets offer little growth opportunity, the preferred strategy is stability or modest growth. The choice of terms is very descriptive; **cows** should be **milked** to generate cash that can be used to support needed investments in stars and question marks.

- **Dogs** are low-market-share businesses in low-growth markets. They do not produce much profit, and they show little potential for future improvement. The preferred strategy for dogs is retrenchment by divestiture.

TOOLS FOR MAKING STRATEGIC DECISIONS

Managers can utilize numerous resources, strategies, and tools for data collection and analysis during the process of formulating strategic decisions. The following sections cover some of the most common and useful aids.

Collecting Data

Data collection and analysis should happen early in the strategic decision-making process. Managers must collect as much information as possible, and then make a timely decision based on the information at hand. Often, healthcare managers have problems with this phase because they mistakenly believe that a magical answer can solve all problems. For example, if your organization cuts your department's budget, as a manager, you may believe that some magical solution can help deal with limited financial resources and somehow make the department staff feel good about the cut. Unfortunately, no right answer exists toward addressing the dilemma imposed by a limited budget.

Managers can also make the mistake of believing that the more time they spend in collecting data, the more accurate their decision will be. Given the high visibility of a manager's position, too much time can be spent collecting information and becoming involved in a research process that instead of signaling a leader may demonstrate a manager who is afraid to make a decision. Not only is this perception extremely harmful to the manager's reputation, but also the manager who spends more time on research than action does not inspire confidence or generate positive results on a consistent basis.

Therefore, remember two important guidelines when collecting data:

- Try to obtain valid, realistic information. Do not expect a one-size-fits-all solution from colleagues or other sources. By recognizing that each situation is unique, a manager brings his or her individual style and approach to problem resolution.

- Recognize that the time frame for making a decision is as important as the decision itself. After you have the information you need, rely on an intelligent gut feeling to arrive at an informed decision. Then initiate the action and begin implementation of your plan.

Studying Established Past Actions

Savvy managers utilize past action—including the actions of predecessors or peer managers—to help formulate new strategies. Assuming someone else's decision was correct, you can gain some insight into your problem and a potential solution. Keep in mind, however, that what worked in the past may not necessarily suit current or future circumstances. Nonetheless, the overall dynamics of the situation may be similar and give you some clue for constructing your own plan of action.

For example, in examining how other managers at your healthcare organizations have responded to budget cuts, you can learn about potential reactions your staff may have toward working with reduced resources. By learning from others' mistakes as well as their positive contributions, you gain insight into what did not work and what did work. In a similar vein, you can ask colleagues for their ideas on what they would do or, better yet, what they did in the past to help staff deal with departmental budget cuts. In both cases, you can find valuable information that provides a strong general frame of reference for formulating your strategy.

Researching Formal References

Formal references are anything that can be construed as **book knowledge**, including journals relevant to your technical area, management texts that offer pragmatic solutions, or your organization's manual of standard operating procedures. Standard operating procedures typically include specific protocols and policies that your organization has adopted or specific bylaws applicable to the situation that you are currently confronting. Peer reviewed journals and other academic publications often can contain a wealth of information. Less used but in some cases more valuable are leadership biographies, both in book form and from business magazines, as these sometimes overlooked sources can have immediately applicable lessons and strategies for a new physician leader. Keeping a notebook handy to jot down ideas, approaches, and **tricks of the trade** in reading such information can help the new physician leader build their own point specific handbook.

Analyzing Hard Data

Hard data can include any information that may have been generated by a questionnaire, form, or survey. Measurable data, or quantitative information, can give you some outlook on the possible impact of your decision. For example, a manager can gather hard data on departmental budget cuts by reviewing organizational history relative to adverse reaction to budget cuts and employee perceptions toward dealing with them. Whether a questionnaire is used or questions are asked informally in a meeting, a survey of staff attitudes to previous budget cuts generates data to assist you in making decisions. (Gathering hard data can also help strengthen the communication link between department colleagues and staff.)

Predicting Advantages and Potential Disadvantages

An important element of data collection is considering the advantages and disadvantages of your options. Who will benefit from your action? How might positive interpersonal effect best be achieved? Also consider when positive results may be realized, and set a time frame of realization of positive output.

Again using the budget-cut example, consider who would be involved with making the budget cuts, when some positive effects could be seen despite the cuts, and what the overall impact of the cuts might be. Set a projected implementation schedule and list the overall benefits, if any, that might emerge from the cuts. At the same time, identify potential negative fallout, including adverse reactions and unfavorable perceptions that may arise. By anticipating negative fallout, you take the first step toward addressing problems and effecting positive action.

Trusting Your Instincts

The final element of data collection is trust in your instincts. Instinctual reaction gives credence to your insight into the problem at hand, the decision you have arrived at, and the action plan you implement. It also mandates a certain amount of introspection—that is, considering the impact a decision will have not only on staff but also on your own activities. Instinctual reaction also means trusting your intelligence and ability to consider the facts objectively, analyze data subjectively, and use common sense to arrive at a course of action.

Analyzing Information

After collecting all significant data, you now must move to the action phase of the decision-making process. This phase entails reviewing all the information collected and setting a course of action and a specific plan for achieving the action. **Action analysis** allows managers to examine the viability of their plans and try to predict whether their decisions are sound and the courses of action will be effective.

Action analysis begins with a data review within the context of four essential factors: the environment, the various functions involved in the action plan, the business consequences of the action taken, and the historical precedent of the action. These four types of analysis allow you to examine every conceivable angle of a decision before taking action.

Environment Analysis

Environment analysis takes into account the theoretical and physical environment in which you operate and the action plan that will be undertaken.

An environment analysis allows managers to look specifically at workplace dynamics while making decisions. The example in Figure 5–2 shows a rehabilitation unit at a metropolitan hospital. The model can

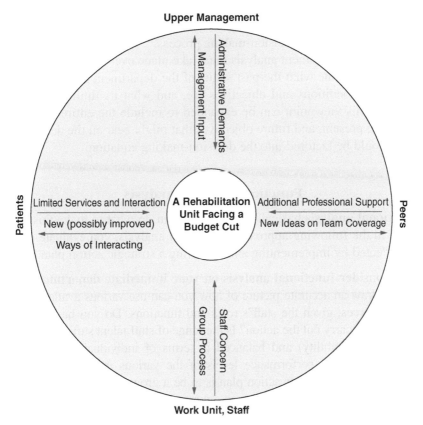

Sphere of influence for a healthcare team facing budget cuts.

FIGURE 5–2. Sphere of influence—planning tool.

assist managers in determining areas that may be most affected by budget cuts, identifying potential areas of concern, and arriving at some suggestions for undertaking the action. Information that is helpful to consider while conducting an environment analysis includes the department's size, the daily volume of patient services, and the revenue the department generates.

Less tangible environmental factors include the prevailing mood of the organization, employee morale in your department, and the administration's attitude toward your department. For example, a department that has direct patient contact traditionally has greater visibility within the organization and consequently gets quicker action and support for carrying out its actions. Hence, as a manager, you must consider your department's status as a factor in your decision-making process.

Finally, environment analysis must take place over a time continuum. Seek to determine what the past status of the department has been, what its present conditions and objectives are, and what its future objectives may be. This viewpoint can be expanded to include the entire organization. Past, present, and future objectives that might bear on the decision at hand should be factored into the decision-making equation.

Functional (Role) Analysis

Functional analysis basically asks, "Who can do what to make this happen?" In the following approach to function analysis, you evaluate every role affected by implementing and executing a strategic action plan.

1. **Consider functional analysis on your immediate department.** Try to draw an accurate picture of how you can use various available staff resources, given the staff's roles and functions. Do you have enough staff to carry out the action? Is the range of staff talent sufficient (eg, in technical ability) and balanced in terms of individual contribution? Consider the performance levels of the various individuals in your department. If your action plan is to be a group process, be certain to include the stronger players on your action team. If significant individual action is required, again consider various individuals' roles, as well as their strengths and weaknesses, and then set your plan accordingly.

2. **Expand the functional analysis to include related departments and colleagues.** For example, a decision you are about to implement may require the support and participation of other departments. You also may need the participation of specialists and other peers within the organization. Try to specify what roles or functions need to be assumed by these individuals and what is required from all participants in installing your plan.

3. **Consider what participation you need from your supervisor.** As your primary mentor, your supervisor is invaluable in guiding you as you implement and execute strategic designs. Also, you may require specific action from a supervisor (eg, influencing another individual within or outside the organization who can further empower your efforts). If you need political clout that only a supervisor can deliver, identify that role during function analysis and enlist participation as appropriate.

4. **Consider benefits to the overall organization.** Detail any specific advantages your organization may enjoy from your strategic decision. Brainstorm any contributions or roles the organization can assume in supporting your decision. Analyze any potential negative impact your decision may have on the organization.

Business Analysis

Before you can fully implement an action plan as a healthcare manager, you must analyze business-related dynamics. First, consider the impact of your decision and its subsequent effect on patients. Specifically, what benefits will patients enjoy? What potential, short-term adverse outcomes may patients endure as a result of your decision?

Two key quality-related themes underlie all aspects of business analysis:

- **Continuous quality improvement (CQI)** should drive all department activities. CQI dictates ongoing quality enhancement as the incentive that fuels everyday activities associated with optimum healthcare delivery.
- **Continuous business development (CBD)** connotes a building-block approach to all departmental activities in management efforts. Every effort undertaken by the department should be done to make the department a stronger, more progressive entity than it was prior to the effort.

Managers reinforce the dynamics of CQI and CBD asking the following questions:

- Will the decision mandate action that is quality conscious?
- Will the decision result in action that improves the quality of services?
- Will the decision initiate action that facilitates departmental mission of progressive development?
- What future departmental or organizational goals may evolve from this decision?
- What will be the ultimate benefit of this action to the patient and the organization?

Finally, in developing a business perspective through analysis, identify any potential negative impacts and business consequences. Specifically, what adverse effect may compromise appropriate use of resources (eg, human, fiscal, and equipment)? Could patients perceive that their welfare is not a top organizational priority? For example, does a construction project severely inconvenience patients? These questions all speak to business dynamics that managers must analyze throughout the decision-making process.

Historical Analysis

Historical analysis takes into account past precedents established in the organization. As a starting point, managers should consider precedents set by past action. What courses of action were taken that were similar in scope to the one you are contemplating?

Managers should review decisions from a political and psychological viewpoint in order to identify possible historical backers and detractors. Healthcare environments are not unlike other corporate cultures in that some individuals look with disdain on certain parts of their organizations. For example, in a metropolitan hospital, the human resource department may be discredited because, according to detractors, it never seems to fill open positions quickly enough. Hence, whenever the human resource department tries to enact a new program, the department experiences a certain resistance from individuals whose positions may be on the line. However, line personnel (such as medical support services) hold human resources in high regard because the department facilitates the training and education that are so vital to the workers' roles. Therefore, enlist the support of potential backers in your decision-making process; they can help sell your new plan.

Healthcare organizations are changing more dramatically and quickly than ever before. In light of ever-escalating competition and a variable fiscal climate, focusing on "how we've always done it before" can under-cut a commitment to presenting new ideas openly and making decisions that explore new frontiers of organizational progress. A commitment to making history is necessary in modern-day health care, where innovative problem solving can mean the difference between success and failure.

Considering Relevance and Contribution to the Organization

After you make a strategic decision and plan a course of action, you should still take time to consider the ramifications of your decisions on the organization, from the perspective of what it can contribute to the organization's goals. By stressing the benefits of your action and gathering the appropriate operational and moral support, you can transform your decision from idea to action.

To crystallize these ramifications, ask yourself the following 10 questions:

1. How do the decision and action enhance the organization's commitment to patients?
2. How do the decision and action reflect the organization's stated values?
3. How do the decision and action contribute to attaining the organization's stated mission?
4. Who should support this decision?
5. Who in the organization will automatically support this decision?
6. How can non-supporters be convinced of the decision's merits and positive contribution to the organization?
7. What are the overall benefits of the action to the organization?
8. How does the decision make the organization better in terms of effectiveness and efficiency?
9. How does my decision make my department a larger contributor to the organizational good?
10. What are two major benefits of this action that everyone in the organization can quickly recognize?

MODELS FOR IMPLEMENTING STRATEGIES AND DECISIONS

Any strategy—no matter how well formulated—can achieve long-term success without proper implementation. In order to successfully put strategies into action, the entire organization and all of its resources must be mobilized in support of them. Mobilizing the organization involves the complete management process—from planning and controlling through organizing and leading.

Common strategic planning pitfalls that hinder implementation include both failures of substance and failures of process:

- **Failures of substance** reflect inadequate attention to the major strategic planning elements—analysis of mission, values and objectives, organizational strengths and weaknesses, and environmental opportunities and threats.
- **Failures of process** reflect poor handling of the strategic planning process itself.

Strategies require supporting structures, well-designed tasks and work-flows, and the right people. And strategies must be enthusiastically supported by leaders who can motivate everyone, build individual performance commitments, and utilize teams and teamwork to best advantage. Only with such total systems support can strategies be implemented well enough to actually achieve competitive advantage. Numerous management consultants and authors have developed models that managers can follow to implement strategic decisions. In addition to the three processes described here, SWOT analysis can also be a useful tool for making and implementing strategic decisions.

Military Model

The military model involves the following 5-part sequence:

1. **Define the objective.** Specify the need or needs and identify the desired outcomes. In defining the objective, identify the optimum outcome and the maximum result that can be achieved.

2. **Identify resources.** Identify all available resources, list their potential contribution to your action, and consider all related resources from other departments within the organization.

3. **Establish the plan.** Write down the specific action you require and establish a time sequence within which the action is needed.

4. **Lay out the course of action.** Set up an incremental plan and establish time checkpoints in which certain objectives should be achieved. For example, if you delegate a particular task to an individual as part of your decision-making and action-execution process, you establish not only a final objective but also interim checkpoints for that individual.

5. **Provide closure.** Closure is made up of those final benchmarks of success that indicate that the plan was successful and the objective reached (such as an accomplished objective or attained goal).

The Parliamentary Model

The parliamentary model is used in many legislative bodies and is similar to the military model in terms of outcomes. The 8-step process is as follows:

1. **Establish need.** Define the needed action and ultimate problem being addressed by the decision and the action taken.

2. **Define the optimum outcome.** What are the best possible results? How can maximum results be achieved by your decision?

3. **Conduct a stakeholder review.** Who is involved? Who has a stake in this action? Who needs to be in on the communication loop?

4. **List pros and cons.** Delineate the positives and negatives of the action taken.

5. **Make an option review.** Review all possible actions and alternative actions.

6. **Review potential consequences.** Consider all adverse reactions to your plan, as well as positive support that might be garnered.

7. **Formulate a step-by-step plan.** Establish a plan and allow for a general preparation and time sequence as evidenced by the information collected in the data-gathering phase and confirmed by continuous contribution and communication with all parties involved.

8. **Analyze achievement.** After you reach the objective, analyze its results, considering the needed action and initial objective. This gives you a reliable measure of success and provides an educational and developmental opportunity for future decisions.

The QUICK Decision Model

In an effort to create an easy-to-remember model that utilizes the best military and parliamentary models (as well as several other less-used models), the authors of this text have devised the QUICK decision model (Figure 5–3). As the name suggests, the method focuses on quickly making decisions and executing action, and it has been used in a number of medical centers as a leadership tool. Each letter of the acronym QUICK

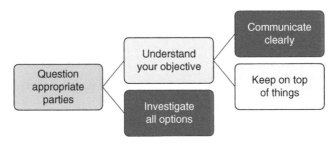

FIGURE 5–3.   The QUICK model.

stands for one of five particular activities that you should do in order to get things done effectively at work:

- Q = Question appropriate parties
- U = Understand your objective(s)
- I = Investigate all options
- C = Communicate clearly to all concerned parties
- K = Keep on top of things, monitoring and reporting progress

SUMMARY

If a healthcare organization does not plan for tomorrow today, it will lose tomorrow. Planning your work and then working plan are not clichés, but must be part of your everyday responsibilities to garner integrity of purpose, cohesion, and progress to your team. Employing the practical strategy of this chapter can help calibrate and guide your efforts to that essential objective.

PRACTICAL RESOURCE—CHAPTER V:
Assessment Tool/Planning Scorecard for Physicians

OVERVIEW

The objective of this tool is to gather personal input as part of our commitment to continually improve our organizational performance to those we serve every day. Physicians play the most important role in our organization's most honorable commitment—providing stellar health care to our community, every day. Accordingly, this questionnaire has been designed specifically to garner individual perspectives and constructive suggestions from all your physicians. It will provide solution-oriented ideas and valuable information for strategic planning.

The executive team must promise complete confidentiality in this process and should use an SSAE attached to this form to collect responses.

Informal feedback sessions should then be held at various facilities to present the scorecard, overall results and responses, and to provide another forum for feedback and solution suggestions.

Organizational Effectiveness

Based on the perspective of your practice, please assign a general rating to the organization/system on the following dimensions using the illustrated scale.

	High				Low
1. Ability to adapt to new demands for medical services	5	4	3	2	1
2. Understanding of change in providing medical services	5	4	3	2	1
3. Active support and professional development of physicians	5	4	3	2	1
4. Keeping everyone informed about new initiatives and programs	5	4	3	2	1
5. Getting input from everyone in an effective manner	5	4	3	2	1
6. Communicating positively to physicians and their office staff	5	4	3	2	1
7. Stressing the benefits of change and progress	5	4	3	2	1
8. Dealing effectively with **negatoid** individuals in the system	5	4	3	2	1
9. Positive and constructive assistance to all practices and individual offices affiliated with SHS	5	4	3	2	1
10. Providing education and expertise needed by office managers	5	4	3	2	1

Additional ideas or insights regarding the overall SHS organization

_____

_____

_____

_____

_____

Customer/Patient Perceptions

Based on your everyday experiences at your office and in your experiences in SHS facilities, how do you believe our patients would rate us on the following issues?

	High				Low
1. Overall quality of care and services	5	4	3	2	1
2. Speed and efficiency of medical care	5	4	3	2	1
3. Compassion and demonstrated caring of staff	5	4	3	2	1
4. Follow-up and supporting action regarding care	5	4	3	2	1
5. Attention to **the little details** involved in care	5	4	3	2	1
6. Effective communication to the patient from the hospital(s), offices, and clinics	5	4	3	2	1
7. Ability to understand the needs of our patients	5	4	3	2	1
8. Adaptability to specific needs of individual patients	5	4	3	2	1
9. Responding with effective solutions to patient needs	5	4	3	2	1
10. Providing **user-friendly** services	5	4	3	2	1

Additional comments and observations regarding patient perceptions

_____

_____

_____

_____

_____

Organizational Profile

Given that all of the following characteristics are relatively important in being a successful physician within the Shore Health System, please select the three factors that you believe are the most critical in your practice and daily responsibilities.

Adaptability, as demonstrated by the ability to respond positively to change, new technology, and increased patient expectations   _____

Accountability, to include personal responsibility and professionalism in every situation   _____

Communication, from listening skills to asking the right questions to presenting information appropriately and effectively   _____

Integrity, consistently forthright and factual in all interpersonal interaction with all members of Shore Health System   _____

Knowledge, the continual pursuit of growth and development activities, and the recognition that every day presents learning opportunities   _____

Independent judgment, the ability to ascertain direction, make key decisions, and set professional goals in a self-reliant (but not self-centered) manner   _____

Professionalism, exemplification of a humanistic commitment, positive outlook, and clear desire toward providing stellar medical service to those in need   _____

Cooperation, highly motivated toward selfless service and maximum support to fellow team members and others intrinsic in the provision of patient care   _____

Perseverance, pursues established course of action patiently and steadfastly in the interest of providing quality care   _____

Innovativeness, apparent in the creative use of available resources and the ability to utilize new, necessary approaches to patient care   _____

Are there other factors that should be included as part of this profile?

_____

_____

_____

_____

_____

Specific Physician Dynamics

Based on your everyday experiences and needs as a physician, please rate the following dynamics based on importance using the scale provided.

	Critical				Low
1. Receptiveness of administration to new ideas and useful suggestions	5	4	3	2	1
2. Administrative corrective action of noted problems and negative issues	5	4	3	2	1
3. Quality and performance of support personnel working at SHS facilities	5	4	3	2	1
4. Training and development support for your office staff	5	4	3	2	1
5. Professional development and management opportunities	5	4	3	2	1
6. Educational opportunities in medicine and specialty areas	5	4	3	2	1
7. Participation in system strategic planning and growth strategies	5	4	3	2	1
8. Clear communication from SHS on new system initiatives and other change dynamics	5	4	3	2	1
9. Quality of information, advertising, and follow-up support with patients	5	4	3	2	1
10. Physician-specific communication, such as a physician-dedicated Web site and CEO forum	5	4	3	2	1

Additional comments and observations regarding your perceptions as an SHS physician

_____

_____

_____

_____

_____

Open Input

Answer the following questions directly and briefly in a list fashion:

1. The best things about practicing as a physician affiliated with SHS are:

a.

b.

c.

2. Three things I'd like to see happen in the near future at SHS and/or in our physician community would be:

a.

b.

c.

3. To be as successful as possible, I need more communication and education regarding:

a.

b.

c.

Any more specific suggestions or additional perspectives

_____

_____

_____

_____

Respondent Data

Please provide the following information:

Job title:

Length of time with our organization as an affiliated physician:

Location/facility:

Please provide the following information if you would like to add further input:

Name:

Phone:

E-mail address:

Thank you for your participation!!!

CHAPTER SIX

Motivation, Communication, and Negotiation

CONTINUOUS LEADERSHIP DEVELOPMENT

Communication is the key to action in building your team and calibrating their efforts toward meaningful, positive action. To ensure that your leadership style develops progressively and your effectiveness grows over time, start with the following strategies:

- **Get as diverse and as much feedback as possible on leadership effectiveness.** Influences on your leadership style can be numerous and diverse; have family, peers, and trusted subordinates give you feedback on your leadership effectiveness. Get suggestions from all these individuals and try to incorporate any good ideas into your future efforts.

- **Give clear direction at all times to all staff members.** Try to specify exactly what is expected and provide as much insight as appropriate on why something should be done. Sharing this information with employees can build trust and allow you to have two-way communication, which is important for a successful leader. Use appropriate follow-up methods to ensure that progress is being made and provide as much additional instruction as possible as employees strive to achieve their goals. Doing so enhances communication and trust, which will be the two most vital components to your success.

- **Give staff an appropriate amount of freedom.** Assume that staff members know what they are doing vital vice until they prove otherwise. Providing too much direction or constraining performance can create the perception that you are unnecessarily overbearing or not trusting your staff. Closely monitor performance, provide inspiration, and measure goal attainment of all staff members.

- **Balance positive and negative information realistically.** You must occasionally give your staff bad news. Provide this information on a timely basis, try to identify an upside (if possible), and deal with problems realistically. On these occasions, verbally stress your confidence that the group can handle adversity and rebound from negative circumstances. Strong leaders participate in adversity as much as in prosperity.

- **Try to keep perspectives on all issues.** The true measure of leaders, in the opinion of many, is their reaction to things that are above and beyond the call of duty or beyond the norm. Try to maintain a balanced view of things, and exhibit the courage and strength necessary to handle tough situations.

- **Learn from every situation.** Health care offers learning opportunities every day. Collect as much information as possible, process that information, and incorporate it into your leadership efforts. Remember that the best way to learn things is to ask appropriate questions. These may be questions that you ask yourself about what you have learned from a situation or questions you ask your peers and your supervisor about their insights and experiences. The more you learn, the greater your frame of reference becomes and the better leader you become.

- **In all cases, be yourself.** Whatever makes sense to you should inspire the judgments you make. Whatever you are comfortable communicating or exhibiting in your words and actions should rule the way you communicate ideas, thoughts, and objectives. Your actions and words are being closely examined by your staff because they provide the impetus and inspiration for staff's activities. Therefore, in the long run, whatever is most natural and comfortable is likely the most progressive precedent to set.

- **Pace your activities both inside and outside the workplace.** Do not try to accomplish everything at once, and make time to enjoy your responsibilities rather than unnecessarily allowing them to be burdensome. Strike a balance between the things that you like to do and the things that you have to do.

- **Trust your instincts.** Your instincts and intelligence are what got you the management job to begin with. As a leader, your good intentions, frame of reference, and basic values are the greatest strengths you have to offer those who want you to succeed. Perhaps the most important point to remember is that the healthcare organization wants you to succeed, your staff wants you to succeed (if for no other reason than it makes their lives easier), and of course you want to succeed. This innate desire, coupled with all the factors discussed throughout this chapter, can allow you to become a strong, positive leader.

BECOMING A TRANSFORMATIONAL LEADER

The term **transformational leadership** is often used to describe someone who uses charisma and related qualities to raise aspirations and shift people and organizational systems into new high-performance patterns. This contrasts with **transactional leadership** in which a leader adjusts tasks, rewards, and structures to help followers meet their needs while working to accomplish organizational objectives (Figure 6–1).

Transactional leadership meets only part of an organization's requirements in today's dynamic environment. A manager must also lead in an inspirational way and with a compelling personality. The transformational leader provides a strong aura of vision and contagious enthusiasm that substantially raises the confidence, aspirations, and commitments of followers. The transformational leader arouses followers to be more highly dedicated, more satisfied with their work, and more willing to put forth extra effort to achieve success in challenging times.

The special qualities that are often characteristic of transformational leaders include

- **Vision:** Having ideas and a clear sense of direction; communicating them to others; developing excitement about accomplishing shared dreams

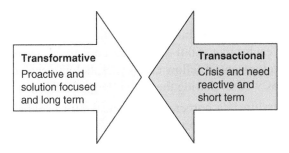

Transformative
Proactive and solution focused and long term

Transactional
Crisis and need reactive and short term

FIGURE 6–1.   Transformative versus Transactional Leadership.

- **Charisma:** Arousing others' enthusiasm, faith, loyalty, pride, and trust in themselves through the power of personal reference and appeals to emotion

- **Symbolism:** Identifying leadership heroes, offering special rewards, and holding spontaneous and planned ceremonies to celebrate excellence and high achievement

- **Empowerment:** Helping others develop, removing performance obstacles, sharing responsibilities, and delegating truly challenging work

- **Intellectual stimulation:** Gaining the involvement of others by creating awareness of problems and stirring their imagination to create high-quality solutions

- **Integrity:** Being honest and credible, acting consistently out of personal conviction, and by following through on commitments

IDENTIFYING APPROPRIATE VALUES

As a healthcare manager, you need to determine which values are important for a healthcare department to maintain and enhance. A logical starting point is to examine the larger organization's values as they are expressed in the mission statement or in other organizational literature.

In general, the following value-based elements should be part of any value-driven healthcare leadership strategy:

- **Care** mandates the provision of health services to patients with the added **human touch** that all staff members should demonstrate when dealing with each patient.

- **Concern** should be shown by the staff not only to patients, but also to each other. Staff should be concerned about the welfare and development of fellow employees, helping each other through crises, as well as sharing the joy of daily victories.

- **Compassion** is a cornerstone of successful healthcare organizations and must be present at all levels of a facility—including your department.

TWO-FACTOR THEORY

Frederick Herzberg's **two-factor theory** offers a now-classic framework for understanding motivation in the workplace. The theory was developed from a pattern identified in the responses of almost 4000 people to questions about work. When questioned about what **turned them on**, respondents tended to identify things relating to the nature of the job itself. Herzberg calls these **satisfier factors**. When questioned about what **turned them off**, they tended to identify things relating more to the work setting. Herzberg calls these **hygiene factors** defined as sources of job dissatisfaction that are associated with critical aspects of job context. These **dissatisfiers** are considered more likely to be a part of the work setting than of the nature of the work itself and can include such things as

- Working conditions
- Interpersonal relations
- Organizational policies and administration
- Technical quality of supervision
- Base wage or salary

Herzberg's two-factor theory argues that improving the hygiene factors, such as by adding piped-in music or implementing a no-smoking policy can make people less dissatisfied with these aspects of their work. But these changes do not in themselves contribute to increase in satisfaction. To really improve motivation, Herzberg advises managers to give proper attention to the satisfier factors.

As part of job content, the satisfier factors deal with what people actually do in their work. By making improvements in what people are asked to do in their jobs, Herzberg suggests that job satisfaction and performance can be raised. Important satisfier factors include

- A sense of achievement
- Feelings of recognition
- A sense of responsibility
- Opportunity for advancement
- Feelings of personal growth

Lately, some scholars have criticized Herzberg's theory as being arcane and difficult to replicate. Yet, as depicted in Figure 6–2, the

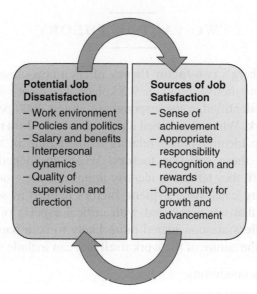

FIGURE 6–2.   The two-factor theory in the healthcare workplace.

two-factor theory remains a useful reminder that there are two important aspects of all jobs in health care:

- **Job content:** What people do in terms of job tasks
- **Job context:** The work setting in which they do it

Furthermore, Herzberg's advice to managers is still timely: (1) Always correct poor context to eliminate actual or potential sources of job dissatisfaction; and (2) be sure to build satisfier factors into job content to maximize opportunities for job satisfaction.

ACQUIRED NEEDS THEORY

David McClelland offers another motivation theory based on individual needs.

- **Need for achievement** is the desire to do something better or more efficiently, to solve problems, or to master complex tasks.
- **Need for power** is the desire to control other people, to influence their behavior, or to be responsible for them.

- **Need for affiliation** is the desire to establish and maintain friendly and warm relations with other people.

According to McClelland, people acquire or develop these needs over time as a result of individual life experiences. In addition, each need carries a distinct set of work preferences. Managers are encouraged to recognize the strength of each need in themselves and in other people. Attempts can then be made to create work environments responsive to them.

People high in the need for achievement, for example, like to put their competencies to work, they take moderate risks in competitive situations, and they are willing to work alone. As a result, the work preferences of high-need achievers include individual responsibility for results, achievable but challenging goals, and feedback on performance.

EXPLORING JOB DESIGN ALTERNATIVES

Job design in many ways is an exercise in **fit**. A good job provides a fit between the needs and capabilities of workers and tasks so that both job performance and satisfaction are high.

To tailor job design to better fit workers' unique abilities and situations, managers can utilize several common job design alternatives, including job simplification, job enlargement and rotation, and job enrichment.

- **Job simplification** involves streamlining work procedures so that people work in well-defined and highly specialized tasks.

Simplified jobs are narrow in job scope, with a limited number and variety of different tasks a person performs. The logic is straightforward: Because some jobs don't require complex skills, workers can be easier and quicker to train, less difficult to supervise, and easy to replace if they leave. Furthermore, because tasks are precisely and narrowly defined, workers can become good at doing the same tasks over and over again.

However, there are some downsides to highly simplified jobs. Productivity can suffer as unhappy workers drive up costs through absenteeism and turnover and through poor performance caused by boredom and alienation. The most extreme form of job simplification is automation or the total mechanization of a job.

The process of job simplification dates back to industrial assembly lines, in which each worker did a specific, simple task to help create a complex product, like an automobile. Today, however, job simplification is less common, particularly in complex healthcare workplaces. In fact, while many healthcare jobs are becoming more complex, some entry-level positions (particularly clerical and technical positions within large healthcare organizations) can still be focused and simplified.

One way to move beyond job simplification is to expand job scope by increasing the number and variety of tasks involved in a job.

- **Job rotation** increases task variety by periodically shifting workers between jobs involving different task assignments.

Job rotation in healthcare settings can include clinical, office, and laboratory settings with a series of functional job stations that workers are assigned to and shuffled on an hourly or daily basis.

- **Job enlargement** increases task variety by combining two or more tasks that were previously assigned to separate workers. The process often involves combining tasks done immediately before or after the work performed in the original job.

Frederick Herzberg questions the value of job rotation and job enlargement. "Why," he asks, "should a worker become motivated when one or more meaningless tasks are added to previously existing ones or when work assignments are rotated among equally meaningless tasks?" By contrast, he says, "**If you want people to do a good job, give them a good job to do.**"

- **Job enrichment** that builds more opportunities for satisfaction into a job by expanding not just job scope but also job depth—that is, the extent to which task planning and evaluating duties are performed by the individual worker rather than the supervisor.

DEALING WITH NONPLAYERS

During the proactive phase of a planned change, managers also need to properly manage **nonplayers**, those team members who do not agree with the change and even work against it. Typically, nonplayers use an assortment of verbal contentious challenges to derail the change process.

Fortunately, proactive managers can respond to common nonplayer complaints effectively as discussed in previous chapters, for example:

Nonplayer's ploy: "That will never work!"

Manager's response: "Well, then tell us specifically what will work."

Nonplayer's ploy: "I have got a problem with this."

Manager's response: "Redefining problems is useless. Give us a solution that might be useful to achieve our goals."

Nonplayer's ploy: "We tried that before, but it did not work."

Manager's response: "We are dealing with the present. How can this work now?"

Nonplayer's ploy: "With all this change, maybe I should find another job."

Manager's response: "I will accept your resignation immediately because change will be constant for years to come in health care."

As these responses indicate, managers can use three principles in managing the nonplayer's resistance.

- **Issue a direct, tactful challenge to the complaining nonplayer.** Do not allow the nonplayer to complain or cast dispersions on group plans without contributing a better idea. The only individual more detrimental to a healthcare organization than a nonplayer in this regard is a manager who allows negativity to become acceptable behavior without holding the nonplayer accountable for constructive contribution, not just destructive criticism.

- **Use plural pronouns, such as we and us.** Doing so encourages the group to recognize that the nonplayer is questioning the entire group's capability, not just yours. This encourages other team members to become accountable for group direction and goal formation, and enlists their participation in countering ill-conceived negativity.

- **Use bottom-line vernacular.** Use words such as useless and immediately, so that the nonplayers are clear in their understanding that game playing, dissention, and group denigration are intolerable when striving for group achievement.

A final component of the proactive stage is your display of natural emotions. Don't be a Pollyanna or Jack Armstrong with an unwarranted positive outlook in the change process; show honest emotion. The group usually recognizes that a manager is in the same boat as they are and will continue to row accordingly.

UNDERSTANDING WHY PEOPLE RESIST CHANGE

Numerous reasons exist for why people in organizations resist planned change. Some of the more common include

- **Disrupted habits:** Feeling upset when old ways of doing things can't be followed
- **Loss of confidence:** Feeling incapable of performing well under the new ways of doing things
- **Loss of control:** Feeling that things are being done to you rather than by or with you
- **Poor timing:** Feeling overwhelmed by the situation or that things are moving too fast
- **Work overload:** Not having the physical or psychic energy to commit to the change

In addition to the preceding, fear is probably the most prevalent emotion cited by healthcare leaders as a major factor in the change process. Nearly everyone experiences uncertainty—fear of the unknown—when they don't understand what is happening or what is coming next.

Another prominent fear for steady players—who often represent the silent majority of a team—is fear of regression. Steady players often view any change with apprehension if the proposed change is not completely presented in a fashion that highlights its improvement value to the status quo. Managers can address fear of regression proactively by recognizing that most steady staff members eventually accept change, provided it is not simply change for the sake of change. As a leader, you have a responsibility to identify how the proposed change brings about new benefits for patients, your organization, your team, and individual team member.

Low-performing staff members—both nonplayers and new, less experienced, and confident employees—often fear having to do more work. Change usually requires increased effort and higher contribution from all staff members. For low-performing staff, increased performance demands are ultimately threatening, because their current level of nonperformance and resistant behavior will be exacerbated by more pressure for optimum performance and an accelerated pace of action. Put bluntly, the need for change presents a great opportunity for low-performing staff to be exposed as incompetent, noncontributory, and detrimental to the provision of stellar health care.

If job descriptions and other substantiating criteria are in place for assessing performance, the change dynamic can provide an excellent opportunity to appraise the low-performing employee's contributions and provide the impetus for termination. This strategy is **rightsizing the right way**, because successful healthcare organizations can only afford to employ individuals who are motivated, competent, and aware that the organization is more important in the work scheme than individual preferences, dissenting opinion, and other **me first** mentalities.

THE POWER OF THANK YOU (FIGURE 6–3)

Perhaps the two most underutilized words at any level of healthcare leadership are **Thank You**. However, these words can realistically and resonantly provide motivation to staff members at any level in a timely and positive manner. If used too often and overemployed, the power of thank you can be compromised by being perceived as redundant and would be diluted from overuse. An example would be profusely thanking an employee for doing something which is part of their normal job responsibilities, as opposed to using it for when the employee truly goes **above and beyond the call of duty**.

There are several nuances to using thank you which will also underscore important themes in a healthcare workplace, as seen in our illustration and outlined below.

1. **Consistency:** To establish consistency of action as an essential workplace value, the phrase **as always** should be linked to the appreciation shown to an employee. For example, if a nurse has gone the extra step to ensure that a child was not fearful of receiving a

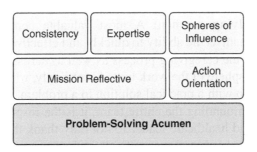

FIGURE 6–3.   The Power of Thank You.

tetanus shot while ensuring that the patient flow in the entire office kept moving, the physician leader can say, "Debbie—great job as always; with your quick and thoughtful action, you made sure that a little kid was not scared and allowed us to take care of all of our patients." It is particularly important in the case of new employees that significant action in this semblance is explained in a manner that helps them understand not only the expectation held in a job position but **why** a particular action and the workplace value that is underscored are vital to the success of the entire operation.

2. **Expertise:** Unique in healthcare workplace is the fact that all staff members have a particular acumen in their field. A skillful leader can adroitly call upon the expertise of each staff member to achieve the desired result. Hence, it is important to underscore the appreciation that the physician leader holds for his/her staff members' expertise by citing it specifically as part of their conveyance of thanks. For example, if a radiology technician has been a particularly stellar analysis of a scan, the physician leader can say, "Thanks much— when we have a complicated case like this, we always look to you as the expert to make sure we get 'the right picture.'"

3. **Excellence:** Outstanding achievement on the part of the staff member should be recognized forthrightly and directly when it occurs. Along with an appropriate citation in the leader's notebook, the healthcare executive should make sure to say thank you **on the spot**, so that the exemplary action is captured is highlighted exactly as that—something which is a great example that should be celebrated and exhibited in full view of the entire staff if possible. Keeping with the leadership principle of always commending outstanding action, the physician leader should employ words such as **outstanding, excellent,** and **remarkable** to highlight significant action and critical contributions among their charges.

4. **Problem-solving acumen:** A most valuable commodity at any healthcare team as the ability to quickly and effectively solve vexing problems in the caregiving process as well as across the span of the operational sphere of the work unit. Accordingly, when a staff member comes up with a practical solution to a problem, particularly one which is confounding the entire team, it is the responsibility of the physician and healthcare leader to not only thank the positive catalyst staff member but also specifically cite as noteworthy the ability to solve problems. This naturally and fluidly reminds all members

of the staff that problem solving based on innovative use of available resources in an efficient and effective manner is rewarded in the workplace and encouraged as a daily responsibility for all members of the team.

5. **Action orientation:** The requisite of taking swift and pertinent action, especially during a crisis (which is at least a once a day event in most healthcare settings) is the characteristic which also should be encouraged through the power of thank you on the part of a physician leader. Outstanding action when confronted by change, conflict, challenge, or crisis based on strong decision making, fortitude, and professional ability is a gold standard in any healthcare team. Healthcare professionals at every level must be certain that when they are charged with taking vital independent action in critical situations, they will be encouraged, supported, and appreciated by their leadership. Thus it becomes particularly important that this is part of the appreciation calculus on the part of the physician leader. The physician leader should cite both the crisis at hand as well as the strategy employed by the superstar who took significant action to **save the day** for the whole team. As is the case with all the strategies in this section, the thanking can be conveyed verbally as well as in written or e-mail fashion; with this particular characteristic, it might be notably worthwhile to send the **action-oriented hero** an e-mail thanking them for their action with a **cc** to your boss as well as a copy for their personnel file in human resources to ensure that the action as noted is part of their work record.

6. **Mission reflective:** All healthcare organizations have a legacy and a lineage within a community which is likely honored by all members of the community as reflected in their continued patronage and support of the healthcare organization or medical practice. A vivid example of this factor would be found in Clara Maass Medical Center in New Jersey which is named after a true healthcare heroine who is a nursing pioneer who literally sacrificed her life in the interest of developing a vaccine for yellow fever. In this case, it is relatively easy for a healthcare leader working at Clara Maass Medical Center to cite a particular action as being reflective of the time-honored mission personified by the self-sacrifice and devotion to duty of their organization's namesake. All healthcare organizations and medical practices have a mission which is usually well publicized and clearly stated to each and every staff member, to include usually a set of values and perhaps in an organizational credo, or a set of beliefs. When thanking

a staff member for extraordinary action which is specifically reflective of the organization's mission, the physician leader should try to specify which one of the values the action reflects when expressing appreciation for the action. For example, the leader can say, "I know it took a lot of time for you to take care of that elderly gentleman who we discharged last week. Not only is patience a virtue, but compassion and commitment to our community members is a major value of our organization; without question, your actions last week in taking care of that gentleman reflected the true compassion and real commitment that we aspire to provide an organization."

7. **Spheres of influence:** As indicated in a previous chapter, there are four sectors of an organization's operating environment which work in confluence every day and consequently can be used in the appreciation communication of a physician leader. To begin with, the patient environment provides bountiful opportunity to cite outstanding action in any circumstance in which a staff member goes the extra step to take care of a patient, which in turn will help flourish the word of mouth reputation of the medical facility. Second, action which reflected credit across the panoply of the organization should be recognized appropriately, as it helps galvanize the operation of the organization and likely contribute to positive morale. Third, selfless actions which help support fellow staff members across the team and group sector within your responsibilities—that is, all of the people who report directly to you—can also be recognized beyond the platitudes of someone simply just being a **good team player**. Finally, individual action which is extraordinary in the way that it helps the individual employee develop and grow on the job while providing a significant contribution to the organizational workflow should be cited in the expression of appreciation.

RESPONDING TO CHANGE RESISTANCE

After a manager recognizes and understands resistance to change, he or she can deal with it in various ways:

- **Education and communication:** Manager uses discussions, presentations, and demonstrations to educate people beforehand about a change.

- **Participation and involvement:** Manager allows others to contribute ideas and help design and implement the change.

- **Facilitation and support:** Manager provides encouragement and training, actively listens to problems and complaints, and helps others to overcome performance pressures.

- **Facilitation and agreement:** Manager provides incentives that appeal to those who are actively resisting or ready to resist. With this approach, the manager typically makes trade-offs in exchange for assurances that change will not be blocked.

- **Manipulation and co-optation:** Manager tries to influence others covertly by providing information selectively and structuring events in favor of the desired change.

- **Explicit and implicit coercion:** Manager forces people to accept change by threatening resistors with a variety of undesirable consequences if they do not go along as planned.

TEAM INTERVENTIONS

Team plays a very important role in organization development. OD practitioners recognize two principles in this respect. First, teams are viewed as important vehicles for helping people satisfy important needs. Second, by improving collaboration within and among teams, organizational performance also improves.

Typically OD interventions designed to improve team effectiveness include

- **Team building:** Structured experiences to help team members set goals, improve interpersonal relations, and become a better functioning team.

- **Process consultation:** Third-party observation and advice on critical team processes (eg, communication, conflict, and decision making).

- **Intergroup team building:** Structured experiences to help two or more teams set shared goals, improve relations, and become better coordinated. Interdependence among all members of the group is essential to achieving change successfully. The following guidelines can help managers and their teams effectively implement change in a cohesive, integrated manner:

o **Identify problems promptly and pragmatically.** Doing so mandates a timely response to cited problems, a practical approach to gathering potential solutions from each staff member, and emphasis on defining new solutions, not reiterating old problems.

o **Elicit solutions from staff members.** Managers must do this constantly and consistently asking all group members, "How can we do X better?"

o **Use interactive feedback.** Present critical information to the group on a timely basis, acknowledge and use suggestive feedback, and reward any new innovations that contribute to the process with group recognition and other appropriate methods.

o **Resolve short-term problems and focus on the long term.** Put the responsibility for a solution on the individuals who identify the problem first, then charge the group with the responsibility of devising a solution that helps make the long-term objective of changing a reality.

o **Reinforce the need for change.** Provide reinforcement throughout the change process by asking team members to help identify new benefits that the change may generate. These benefits can be any advantages the organization, department, or individual may realize that were not identified initially but are now readily apparent and tangible for the group to identify and discuss.

o **Cite examples of positive change.** Whenever possible, link past examples of positive group change and current challenges. You probably can easily identify a past action that was so daunting that by comparison a current change project is seemingly easy.

DEALING WITH STRESS

In a healthcare setting, the jobs that people perform—and the relationships and circumstances under which they have to do them—are often causes of significant stress. Formally defined, **stress** is a state of tension experienced by individuals facing extraordinary demands, constraints, or opportunities.

Any look toward a healthcare career is incomplete without considering stress as a challenge that you are sure to encounter along the way—and a challenge you must be prepared to help others learn to deal with.

Sources of Stress

The things that cause stress are called **stressors**. Whether stressors originate directly in the work setting or emerge in personal and nonwork situations, they all have the potential to influence work attitudes, behavior, and job performance (Figure 6–4).

Work factors have an obvious potential to create job stress. Some 46% of workers in one survey reported that their jobs were highly stressful; 34% said that their jobs were so stressful that they were thinking of quitting. Today, most workers experience stress in long hours of work, excessive e-mails, unrealistic work deadlines, difficult bosses or coworkers, and unwelcome or unfamiliar work. Stress is also associated with excessively high- or low-task demands, role conflicts or ambiguities, poor interpersonal relations, or career progress that is too slow or too fast. Stress tends to be high during periods of work overload, when office politics are common, and among people working for organizations undergoing staff cutback and downsizing. (This latter situation and lack of **corporate loyalty** to the employee can be especially stressful to employees who view themselves as **career** employees and who are close to retirement age.)

A variety of personal factors are also sources of potential stress for people at work. Such individual characteristics as needs, capabilities, and

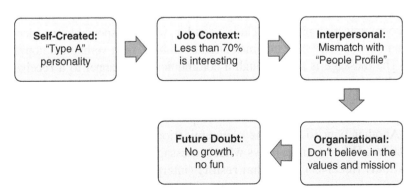

FIGURE 6–4.   Sources of Negative Stress.

personality can influence how one perceives and responds to work situations. Researchers, for example, identify a **type A personality** that is high in achievement orientation, impatience, and perfectionism. Type A people are likely to create stress in circumstances that others find relatively stress free. Type A people, in a sense, bring stress on themselves. Stressful behavior patterns of Type A personalities include

- Always moving, walking, and eating rapidly
- Acting impatient, hurrying others, disliking waiting
- Doing, or trying to do, several things at once
- Feeling guilty when relaxing
- Trying to schedule more in less time
- Using nervous gestures such as a clenched fist
- Hurrying or interrupting the speech of others

Finally, stress from nonwork factors can have spillover effects on an individual's work. Stressful life situations, including such things as family events (eg, the birth of a child), economics (a sudden loss of extra income), and personal affairs (a preoccupation with a bad relationship), are often sources of emotional strain. Depending on the individual and his or her ability to deal with them, preoccupation with such situations can affect one's work and add to the stress of work-life conflicts.

COMMUNICATION ESSENTIALS

Formally defined, **communication** is an interpersonal process of sending and receiving symbols with messages attached to them. The key elements in the communication process include a **sender**, who is responsible for encoding an intended message into meaningful symbols, both verbal and nonverbal. The message is sent through a communication channel to a **receiver**, who then decodes or interprets its meaning. This interpretation may or may not match the sender's original intentions. **Feedback**, when present, reverses the process and conveys the receiver's response back to the sender.

Another way to view the communication process is as a series of questions. **Who?** (sender) **says what?** (message) **in what way?** (channel) **to whom?** (receiver) **with what result?** (interpreted meaning).

Effective communication occurs when the intended message of the sender and the interpreted meaning of the receiver are one and the same.

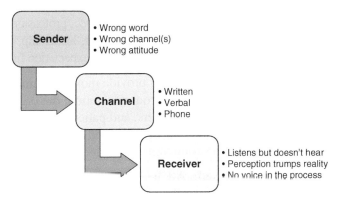

FIGURE 6–5.   Negative Communication Stress.

Although this may seem like the goal in any communication attempt, it is not always achieved. Efficient communication occurs at minimum cost in terms of resources expended, such as the amount of time involved. Efficiency is one reason why so many people rely on voice mail and e-mail, rather than visiting others personally to communicate a message.

Efficient communication is not always effective and can fall into the category of a negative work stress element rapidly (Figure 6–5). A low-cost approach such as an e-mail note to a distribution list may save time, but it does not always result in everyone getting the same meaning from the message. Without opportunities to ask questions and clarify the message, erroneous interpretations are possible. By the same token, an effective communication may not always be efficient. If a manager visits each team member individually to explain a new change in office procedures, this process may guarantee that everyone truly understands the change. But it may also be very costly in the demands it makes on the manager's time. A team meeting is more efficient. In these and other ways, potential trade-offs between effectiveness and efficiency must be recognized in communication.

Identifying Communication Sources

Two types of communication are important to all members of healthcare teams, especially managers:

- **Incoming communication** includes directives, mandates, directions, guidance, support, feedback, questions, consultation, advice, demands, and expectations.

- **Outgoing communication** includes compliance, professional development, action, growth, support, team insight, leadership, contribution and expertise, and finally satisfaction and expectation fulfillment.

For healthcare managers, six sources provide most incoming communication and are the target of outgoing communication: the organization, supervisors, family and friends, staff, peers, and patients.

Additionally, communication can be classified by the source of the message. Some of the common communication sources include

- **The organization itself:** All healthcare organizations generate directives to managers regarding how to manage staff, the ways to conduct technical activities, and the quality of contributions expected from staff. These directives may be presented in written or oral form, and the information may be implicit or explicit. For example, an implicit directive may be that you maintain the highest moral and ethical standards in the delivery of your particular segment of healthcare service. However, if this directive is written into the organization's code of conduct, its mission statement, or a set of organizational standards, it is explicit. Additionally, newsletters, annual reports, newspaper articles, and other sources of information can clarify the values of a healthcare organization.

- **Supervisors:** Your manager provides you with a certain amount of direction in how to conduct your job. This direction may include a history of departmental responsibilities, background into the department's prior performance, or some insight into individual members. Supervisors also should provide a set of detailed expectations they hold for your department.

- **Family and friends:** The demands of a healthcare management job pretty much dictates a leader's working hours. For example, if an emergency requires your presence, most likely you will be there—even if it is your scheduled day off or hours past the end of your shift. Being a manager can put a strain on personal relationships, and family and friends may have difficulty adjusting to healthcare management work hours. Take a proactive, rather than reactive, approach to this potential problem. From the start, orient family and friends to the realities and expectations of your job. Remind them that a healthcare management job is not a 9-to-5 position; rather, job demands are the primary determinants of your working hours. Above all, keep communication constant and open between with your family and friends.

- **Staff:** As a manager, you seek and receive feedback from your staff on a variety of issues. Feedback can include technical issues involving your department, individual concerns relative to the job, and suggestions on improving performance across the department. Conversely, as a manager, share information as appropriate with your staff and get their input and suggestions. This vital exchange can help you form a progressive frame of reference for dealing with management issues. For example, suppose your organization plans to implement a bonus-incentive compensation system. After attending several management meetings on this issue, you are curious about employees' reaction to the new program. You may choose to discuss the issue in a department meeting, in one-on-one meetings with key employees, or informally within the context of ongoing discussions with staff. These communication efforts can give you a frame of reference that you can then use in your management discussions to help further refine the bonus-incentive compensation system within the organization.

- **Peers and colleagues:** Peers and colleagues—that is, fellow managers—rely on you to provide technical expertise in key areas. In exchange, they provide their technical expertise and real-life management experiences to you, when appropriate.

- **Patients:** The most important source of incoming information is the patient. In a sense, healthcare managers receive all communications from patients—or at least are party to all communications. Managers must take the lead in answering patients' requests, handling their complaints, and incorporating their input into the general management strategy of patient service. For example, the manager of a physical rehabilitation department of a small hospital may receive specific complaints or compliments about the way physical therapy was provided for a particular patient. However, the same patient may also comment on the hospital's billing system, its parking facilities, or how cooperative the security and reception personnel were in helping the patient find your department. All feedback—both positive and negative—should be incorporated into a manager's ongoing notes and relayed to appropriate individuals within the organization.

Figure 6–6 provides some easy to understand but sometimes difficult to maintain **stress busters** relative to the above.

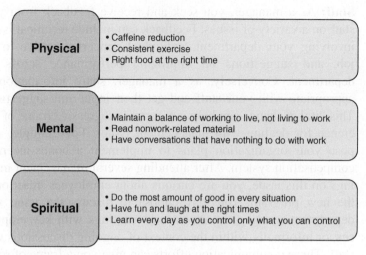

FIGURE 6–6.   Stress Busting Strategies.

Making Successful Presentations

Presentations are a frequent responsibility for healthcare managers. Audiences for presentations can be your team, your peers, your supervisors, or perhaps a combination of all three groups.

Keep the following strategies in mind to make presentations as successful as possible:

- **Be prepared.** Know what you want to say; know how you want to say it; and rehearse saying it.

- **Set the right tone.** Give the audience your complete focus—make eye contact and be pleasant, confident, and engaging.

- **Organize your message into points.** State your purpose, make important points, follow with details, and then summarize.

- **Support your points.** Give specific reasons for your points and state them in understandable terms.

- **Accent the presentation.** Use good visual aids and provide supporting handouts when appropriate.

- **Add the right amount of polish.** Attend to the details, such as having the room, materials, and other arrangements ready to go.

- **Check your technology.** Check everything ahead of time. Make sure it works and know how to use it.

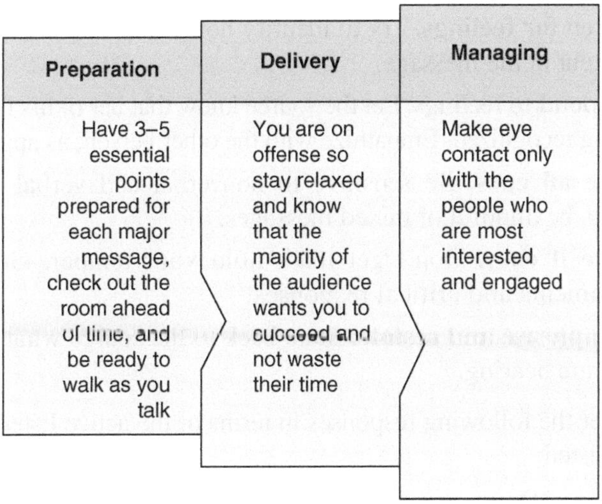

Preparation	Delivery	Managing
Have 3–5 essential points prepared for each major message, check out the room ahead of time, and be ready to walk as you talk	You are on offense so stay relaxed and know that the majority of the audience wants you to succeed and not waste their time	Make eye contact only with the people who are most interested and engaged

FIGURE 6–7.   Presentational Keys.

- **Don't bet on the Internet.** Beware of plans to make real-time Internet visits during a presentation. Save Web site and other content on a disk or your hard drive and then use a browser to open the file.

Figure 6–7 provides a set of critical keys for preparing and delivering presentations that augment this information.

Active Listening

When people talk, they are trying to communicate something. That **something** may or may not be what they are saying. **Active listening** is the process of helping the source of a message say exactly what he or she really means. Active listening requires considerable effort, but the effects on the communication process can be beneficial.

Keep in mind the following guidelines for active listening:

- **Stop talking.** You can't listen if you're talking.
- **Show that you want to listen.** Remove any potential distractions, and try to physically put the other person at ease.
- **Listen for message content.** Try to hear exactly what content is being conveyed in the message.

- **Listen for feelings.** Try to identify how the source feels about the content in the message.
- **Respond to feelings.** Let the source know that her or his feelings are being recognized. Empathize with the other person, as appropriate.
- **Note all cues.** Be sensitive to nonverbal and verbal messages. Also, be mindful of mixed messages.
- **Take it easy.** Don't get mad; hold your temper. Go easy on arguments and critical responses.
- **Paraphrase and restate.** State back to the source what you think you are hearing.

Consider the following responses in terms of the active listening ideals previously listed:

Question: "Don't you think employees should be promoted on the basis of seniority?"

Passive listening response: "No, I don't!"

Active listening response: "It seems that's your opinion. Tell me why."

Question: "What does the supervisor expect us to do about these out-of-date computers?"

Passive listening response: "Do the best you can, I guess."

Active listening response: We are all aware of the existing hardware problems. As our expert in this area, please give us two new ideas on software solutions to our common problem. After all, each of us is responsible to all of us.

The preceding examples show how active listening can facilitate and encourage communication in difficult circumstances, rather than discourage it.

Negotiating

What strategies would you use if:

- you have been offered a promotion and would really like to take it, but the pay raise offered is less than you hoped?
- you have enough money to order one new computer for your department, but you have requests for two new machines?

These are examples of the many situations in today's healthcare workplace that involve **negotiation,** the process of making joint decisions when the parties involved have different preferences. People negotiate over such diverse matters as salary, merit raises and performance evaluations, job assignments, work schedules, work locations, special privileges, and many other considerations. All such situations are susceptible to conflict and require exceptional communication skills.

Most new physician leaders are not born negotiators, skilled negotiators, or educated negotiators. Few healthcare curriculums offer courses of practicum experiences on negotiating. And yet, in the course of a given day, healthcare managers may negotiate a fee-for-services contract, establish new performance standards for a nonperforming employee, or set a new schedule for an operating room. All these interactions, like many of the interpersonal interactions managed by an effective physician leader, call for negotiation skill, strategy, and savvy.

This section, although hardly exhaustive, offers an overview of the negotiation process, as well as some basic strategies that healthcare managers can implement into their daily managerial duties.

Choosing a Negotiation Approach

In general, two types of goals exist in the world of negotiation:

- **Substance goals** are concerned with outcomes. They are tied to the **content** issues of the negotiation.

- **Relationship goals** are concerned with processes. They are tied to the way people work together while negotiating and how they (and any constituencies they represent) will be able to work together again in the future.

Negotiation can be considered successful when issues of substance are resolved and working relationships among the negotiating parties are maintained or even improved.

The way each party approaches a negotiation can have a major impact on its outcomes.

- In **distributive negotiation**, each party makes claims for certain preferred results. This is a competitive win-lose approach in which one party can gain only if the other loses. Relationships are often sacrificed as the negotiating parties focus only on their respective self-interests.

- In **principled negotiation**, a win-win orientation operates. The interests of all parties are considered, and the goal is to base the final outcome on the merits of individual claims. Everyone looks for ways for all claims to be satisfied if possible, with no one **losing** in the process.

Many healthcare managers approach negotiation as a series of appeals that they make to the other party. Although appeals can be an effective way of gaining your opponent's attention, appeals alone are not typically enough to reach a win-win agreement.

Essentially, negotiating appeals fall into the following basic types:

- **Appeal to ego:** A negotiator uses an array of compliments, ego stroking, and other self-esteem gratification techniques to reach a favorable settlement. Using expressions like **a smart individual like you, someone who is a real go-getter**, or **an intelligent manager like yourself**, as preambles to statements helps to build an appeal-to-ego strategy. This strategy may be effective in the short term, but over the long term it can be seen as manipulative, less than genuine, and basically phony.

- **Appeal to authority:** In this case, an individual uses an authority such as a state regulation board, the board of directors, or other proverbial **powers that be** as the driving factor in why a negotiation settlement should be reached quickly and favorably. This tactic is not only somewhat disingenuous, as it connotes a power play by the negotiator who uses it, but is also an abdication of authority relative to the basic responsibility of the individuals present at the negotiation table.

- **Appeal to the norm:** This appeal is in evidence when a negotiator cites the need for commonality or normalcy as a driving force for reaching a settlement. Statements such as **most physicians would take this deal** or **every hospital in the state does it** are examples of appeal-to-norm strategies. This technique may be effective in some cases, where standards and practices are the prominent features of the need to reach a negotiated settlement, but in all cases it is a less-than-effective strategy.

- **Appeal to emotion:** Anger, pride, friendship, gravity (such as **if we don't do this, the hospital will close!**), and other emotional drivers are used to trigger a negotiated settlement in an appeal-to-emotion ploy. Appealing to emotion is a perilous tactic for a healthcare leader to use. Fundamentally, most people who have had any sort of tenure in health care have witnessed a wide array of emotionalism displayed by patients and employees on any given day. Therefore, they are not likely to be motivated by someone crying, yelling, threatening, conjoining, or displaying any other type of emotional behavior that is not specifically related to the negotiation objective at hand.

- **Appeal to a vision:** Here, a negotiator presents a picture of what the final negotiating outcome may be. Appealing to a vision is perhaps the only effective strategy among the appeal-process negotiation techniques. In painting a picture of a harmonious workplace, effective emergency room, progressive medical service organization, or any other favorable vision of healthcare excellence, a negotiator can create a vision that is equally alluring to their opponent as to themselves. The vision can be not only the objective for the negotiation but also the driving motivation for reaching a settlement. However, the vision must be one that is equally shared and desired by both negotiation parties; otherwise, the tactic is doomed to fail.

- **Appeal to mission:** A negotiator constantly cites the mission of the healthcare organization as the driving force for reaching a negotiated settlement. This can be an effective appeal only if coupled with the vision appeal and other artful negotiation.

- **Appeal to personal relationships:** Friendship, collegiality, past history, and other personal notes are used as catalysts for obtaining a progressive settlement. Though a certain amount of strength of interpersonal relationship can be drawn on in any negotiation, the effective negotiator does not rely strictly on personal friendship as the centerpiece for negotiation. Simply put, if an individual uses personal friendship as a mainstay of negotiation, the opponent can simply say something along the lines of "Friendship is one thing, business is another—let's get down to the brass tacks of reaching a good agreement."

Many elements of the psychological win-win approach can be incorporated into a more effective strategy of the **mutual benefit logical approach** to negotiation.

The mutual benefit logical approach is based on several basic beliefs:

- **Preparation is key.** If you are prepared and your opponent is not, or is not as well prepared as you are, the odds increase in your favor that you can prevail in the negotiation. Preparation takes several forms in logical negotiation: knowing your opponent, preparing your bargaining position, preparing counterarguments, and planning overall negotiation strategies are all examples of well-prepared negotiation techniques.

- **Knowledge of your opponent is crucial.** By understanding your opponent's position, analyzing potential methods and approaches of your opponent, and counteracting your opponent's forays in the negotiation process, the likelihood of a negotiation victory is enhanced. Again, preparation is key, and the requirement that the negotiator does the homework is paramount to success.

- **Establish a negotiation range.** Prepared negotiators understand the differences between wants and needs and negotiate by focusing on needs. Often, negotiating parties reach an immediate impasse because both sides endeavor to move the other party toward the **want** position. By focusing on needs, there exists the opportunity for a well-negotiated settlement that can be favorable to both parties.

Knowing an Opponent's Position

At the outset of the negotiation process, a savvy negotiator tries to ascertain his or her opponent's position. This can be achieved by asking your opponent to prioritize the list of most important agenda items for the negotiation. You can then ascertain the primary and secondary agenda items for your opponent. Furthermore, try to determine the strategic position of your opponent on mutually beneficial needs range. By asking a sequence of questions, you can elicit more specific information about your opponent's desired outcomes for the negotiation.

The following questions force your opponent to be more specific about his or her position:

- What do you need to have happened here at the negotiation table?
- Specifically what do you need from our discussions?
- Why is this particular initiative important to you?
- Which one of these items is the most important to you?
- What are you looking for from this negotiation?
- Would you please list for me—so we all understand—what your priorities are, listed in numerical order?
- What do you need to get done here at the negotiating table, or what do we need to get done?
- What do you want to get done, or what do we want to get done here at the table? (Note: By using this and the preceding question in concert, you may be able to get a sense of an opponent's **dream objective**.)

- How can we make this happen?
- Can you directly, honestly, and specifically tell us what your ultimate objectives are for this negotiation?

In seizing the initiative in trying to unveil your opponent's position, you are better prepared to list priorities for the negotiation and identify not only the primary and secondary needs of the opponent, but your potential trade-off positions for the negotiation. Once again, by simply being prepared and taking a proactive stance in the negotiation process, you gain an upper hand that helps facilitate a more favorable result to the negotiation process.

Avoiding Negotiating Pitfalls

The negotiation process is admittedly complex. Negotiators must guard against several common mistakes. Many obstacles can stand in the way of success in reaching an agreement.

Pitfalls such as the following can too easily create win-lose situations, which can ultimately result in poor final results:

- **The myth of the fixed pie:** When you fall prey to this pitfall in negotiation, you assume that in order for you to gain, the other person must give up something. Negotiating this way fails to recognize the possibility that sometimes the pie can be expanded or utilized to everyone's advantage.
- **Nonrational escalation of conflict:** In this pitfall, the negotiator becomes committed to previously stated demands and allows concerns for ego and face-saving to increase the perceived importance of satisfying these demands.
- **Overconfidence and ignoring the others' needs:** The error here is becoming overconfident that your position is the only correct one and failing to see the needs of the other party and the merits in its position.
- **Too much telling, too little hearing:** When committing a telling problem, you don't really make yourself or your side understand. When committing a hearing problem, you don't listen sufficiently to understand what the other is saying.

Reaching Agreement

At a certain point—a point that is difficult to define because each negotiation is different—you should move to close the deal.

Generally, you would want to close the deal when you have ascertained that your opponent has reached a position of agreement with you within the mutually beneficial need range that is amenable to both parties.

At that point, you can choose among the following options:

- Verify the position of both parties.
- Take the deal.
- Reject the deal.
- Consider the long-range ramifications of accepting or rejecting the deal.
- Consider alternative deals with other parties.
- Reevaluate the benefits provided by the impending deal.
- Perhaps most important, listen to and trust your gut, and gauge your comfort level with the deal.
- Summarize and reiterate the tenets of the deal so that both parties understand.

If the answers to all the items on this checklist are relatively positive, you should embrace the deal that has been generated through the negotiation strategy. Unfortunately, it may not always be possible to achieve integrative agreements. When negotiations reach the point of impasse, dispute resolution through mediation or arbitration can be useful.

- **Mediation** involves a neutral third party who tries to improve communications between negotiating parties and keep them focused on relevant issues. This mediator does not issue a ruling or make a decision, but can play an active role in discussions. Mediation often includes making suggestions in an attempt to move the parties toward agreement.

- **Arbitration** is a stronger form of dispute resolution. Arbitration involves a neutral third party, the arbitrator, who acts as a judge and issues a binding decision. The arbitration process usually includes a formal hearing in which the arbitrator listens to both sides and reviews all facets of the case before making a ruling.

As in all leadership endeavors, no right or wrong answers exist in the negotiation process. However, by following the introductory guidelines in this chapter—and more important, trusting your intrinsic intelligence and negotiation savvy—the art of mutually beneficial negotiation is well within your grasp as a healthcare manager.

PRACTICAL RESOURCE—CHAPTER VI:
Criterion-Based Performance Evaluation

PART I: INSTRUCTIONAL BOOKLET

Overview

This performance evaluation system is designed to provide all organizational members with meaningful insight into their individual performance and to properly reward performance through our merit compensation system. It is the responsibility of both the organizational member and the manager to participate actively in the process by examining **job performance**, **how** we do our job, and **significant additional action** we contribute in providing top quality health care to our community.

The instructions contained in this booklet are supplemented with brief guidelines on the form. All managers attend educational sessions on completing and delivering the appraisal, and human resource staff is available to assist you in this important responsibility.

SECTION I: Administrative Data

The first section of the form requires the entry of employee data, most of which is contained in the employee's personnel file. The space provided for **reviewing manager** should indicate the individual responsible for the review and to whom the subject employee directly reports. **Salary grade** information may be completed by utilizing the designated code or range as indicated in the personnel file.

The last entry in this section refers to the evaluation occasion and should be completed as follows:

- **Annual** would indicate the normal, once-a-year performance review to be completed on the employee's anniversary date in the current position.
- **Initial orientation** would indicate the review conducted with a newly hired employee at the first 3-month anniversary of employment or after 3 months in a new position.
- **Redirective probationary** should be utilized 3 months after any review which does not meet the minimum standard for performance (as indicated by a total evaluation score of <250 points).
- **Transfer/promotion** should be used prior to the transfer or promotion of an employee. This evaluation would reflect less than 1 year of performance and could be incorporated into the annual review.

SECTION II: Job Responsibilities

This section facilitates a review of the major responsibilities of the organizational member's job. The job responsibility should be considered, along with any goals and objectives of significant scope that were assigned at the start of the review period. The total number of major responsibilities should not exceed 10 in total, and each should be assigned a performance value using a multiple of 5 (refer to the instructions in Appendix A of this guidebook for specific instructions on determining and assigning the performance value). The performance value total will be 100.

Following the establishment of the job responsibilities and related performance values, the reviewing manager should enter the responsibilities and their respective performance values into the designated spaces on Section II of the performance evaluation form. The manager should then place a rating, based on documented evaluated performance, for each job responsibility using the following scale:

1. Below expectation/substandard performance consistently demonstrated
2. Meets expectation/standard performance consistently demonstrated
3. Exceeds expectation/outstanding performance consistently demonstrated

Determining the Performance Value

The **performance value** for each particular job responsibility should take into consideration both the time quotient and weighted value relative to the job responsibility. The **time quotient** is the normal amount of time usually applied to performing the job responsibility. The **weighted value** reflects the relative importance of the responsibility to the overall job position.

To determine the performance value, the manager should list all the major job responsibilities in the column designated, with no more than 10 entries. The manager should then reflect the normal amount of time spent in each responsibility utilizing multiples of 5. Then, considering the overall importance of the job responsibility to the work role, a weighted value should be entered, again using multiples of 5 in the column designated.

The time quotient and weighted value will often be identical. However, certain job responsibilities can have different time quotients and weighted values due to specific employee expertise, the nature of the responsibility, and other nuances. The manager has the latitude to assess each responsibility from both a time quotient and weighted value perspective.

The overall sum of both the time quotient column and the weighted value column will each be 100.

The performance value is then reached by adding the time quotient and weighted value for each responsibility and then dividing by 2. The performance value should then be entered in the designated column, and the total of all performance values will naturally total 100.

Performance value worksheet			
POSITION			
Job responsibility	Time quotient	Weighted value	Performance value
1			
2			
3			
4			
5			
6			
7			
8			
9			
10			
Totals			

The manager should then multiply the performance value for each component by the corresponding rating for each component to compute the overall score for that job component. Accordingly, the maximum score for this section will be 300.

The responsibilities of each manager are as follows:

- Document performance continuously throughout the course of the evaluation period.

- Rate each reporting staff member individually and fairly.

- Consider each job responsibility independently and comprehensively.

- Review all significant aspects of performance and reflective indicators in determining ratings.

Comments can be placed in the designated area and the total score should be placed in the space provided by simply adding all of the scores in the **score** column.

SECTION III: The CARE Factors

Our organization is resolute in its commitment toward providing those needing our services with health care reflecting dedication to our community, allegiance to all organizational members and our mission, responsiveness to student needs and excellence of education. This section gives the manager the opportunity to assess the employee in these vital areas and provides the employee with a forthright assessment of the quality of their professional performance.

As illustrated in Section III, each element of the CARE Formula is augmented by 5 factors. These factors are defined in the management texts provided in our organization's management training. Each individual component should be graded using the following scale:

5	4	3	2	1
Outstanding	Above average	Satisfactory	Marginal	Unsatisfactory

Each factor should be scored accordingly and applicable comments should be entered in rating outstanding or unsatisfactory performance. Comments should be supplemented using criteria from the management texts.

SECTION IV: Significant Action/Critical Contribution

This section is to cite performance which is special in nature and is not reflected in Section II as a normal job component. Any applicable action must be substantiated by the use of at least one of the following reflective codes. Each code citation merits 5 points. One action might mandate more than 1 code, meriting a score derived by assigning 5 points to each designation. If the individual missed an opportunity to make a critical contribution, the action should be notated here with no points assigned. The absolute maximum for this section is 100 points.

Code	Action description
A	Performance which is clearly **above and beyond the call of duty** in which an employee responded in a substantiated stellar fashion
B	A major cost-saving program or initiative implemented by an employee
C	New program implementation by an employee in which a measurable performance benefit was realized
D	Time efficiency as produced by an employee-generated initiative or program implementation
E	Operational improvement, such as a procedure upgrading or new system approach which significantly improves operational flow
F	Major quality improvement which has a marked benefit to users and adds to the organization's overall quality improvement process
G	Undertaking of new responsibilities created by unforeseen circumstances such as turnover, crisis, expansion, etc
H	Productivity enhancements, such as new programs, inventions, innovations, or other creations which spark increased productivity
I	Human resource maximization, where the employee has devised a new strategy for optimizing staff performance and contribution
J	Positive reaction to a major, unforeseen negative crisis which taxed the entire work unit and to which the employee responded notably
K	Undertaking of a new, major project or program not assigned at the start of the performance review period
L	Major development activities which increase the employee's professional expertise as well as their contribution to the organization

SECTION V: Training and Development Plan

The continuous professional development of every organizational member is essential to our success and progressive growth. This section should contain developmental activities that will enhance the organizational member's skills and expertise. These suggestions should be considered with input from the organizational member and can include in-service programs, cross-training, formal training and educational programs, and any other applicable developmental strategy.

SECTION VI: Comments, Overall Rating, and Signatures

This section is very straightforward. The employee's comments can be written in the space provided, with additional pages attached if necessary. The manager's comments can be written in the space provided to amplify or further illustrate the employee's scope of performance. The 3 requisite signatures (the organizational member, the manager, and the reviewing manager) should be affixed in the spaces provided.

Finally, an overall tally of the rating numbers should be entered in the space designated, with an overall maximum of 500 points possible.

Section I: Administrative Data
Performance evaluation form
Employee's Name:
Organizational Start Date:
Positional Start Date:
Reviewing Manager/Supervisor:
Department:
Date of Last Evaluation:
Date of This Evaluation:
Salary Grade or Range:
Evaluation Occasion: ☐ Annual ☐ Initial ☐ Orientation ☐ Redirective ☐ Probationary ☐ Transfer/Promotional

Section II: Position Responsibilities

Enter each position responsibility, its respective performance value, and a rating and overall score in the spaces indicated. Total the overall scores, and enter the sum in the designated space.

Job responsibility	Performance value	Rating	Score	Comments
1				
2				
3				
4				
5				
6				
7				
8				
9				
10				
Total score				

Section III: The CMI CARE Factors

Rate each factor using the numerical scale. Total all scores and enter the page total in the space provided.

Part A: Community   **Comments**

Commitment	5	4	3	2	1
Decency	5	4	3	2	1
Employer-Peer Relations	5	4	3	2	1
Fortitude	5	4	3	2	1
Perceptiveness	5	4	3	2	1

Part A Total: _____

Part B: Allegiance   **Comments**

Communication	5	4	3	2	1
Cooperation	5	4	3	2	1
Delegation	5	4	3	2	1
Integrity	5	4	3	2	1
Perseverance	5	4	3	2	1

Part B Total: _____

Part C: Responsiveness   **Comments**

Energy Level	5	4	3	2	1
Independent Judgment	5	4	3	2	1
Industry	5	4	3	2	1
Planning	5	4	3	2	1
Professional Bearing	5	4	3	2	1

Part C Total: _____

Part D: Excellence   **Comments**

Accountability	5	4	3	2	1
Adaptability	5	4	3	2	1
Creativity	5	4	3	2	1
Knowledge	5	4	3	2	1
Technical Expertise	5	4	3	2	1

Part D Total: _____

Section III Total: _____

Section IV: Significant Action/Critical Contribution

Cite any positive significant action and critical contributions by the employee during the review period, as per the guideline code system.

Significant action/ critical contribution	Code and total points for positive action	Comments

Section V: Training and Development Plan

List all activities the employee should undertake in the next review period to enhance performance and professional expertise.

Activity	Benefit to employee growth	Plan/timing

Section VI: Comments, Overall Rating, and Signatures		
Employee comments:	Overall rating	Score
	Section II	
	Section III	
	Section IV	
	Total	
Manager/supervisor comments:	Employee's signature	Date
	Manager's signature	Date
	Reviewing manager's signature	Date

CHAPTER SEVEN

Maximizing Team Action and Individual Performance

Regardless of their experience or rank within the organization, the task of synergizing individual talents into a larger group effort is often problematic for new healthcare manages. Building a team can be a complex task. Trying to establish common goals, objectives, and shared dedication to a mission is one thing—managing and harnessing the abilities and talents of a diverse group of individuals so as to move toward a mutual goal is another thing altogether. If you examine the overall structure of your healthcare organization, you will probably find it consisting of many solid teams. Some departments may be stronger than others—perhaps their members have stronger talents or maybe they work together more smoothly and efficiently. If the department is considered to be a stellar team, it probably has both these elements of talent and group cohesion. As a newly appointed healthcare manager, you can establish a strong team orientation with these resonant and resilient components.

This chapter will discuss ways of analyzing a team and determining the potential contribution of each member to the team effort. After analyzing the work personality as it relates to health care, the chapter will close with a detailed discussion on establishing and then reinforcing a value-driven team orientation. Upon reviewing these concepts and considering their potential application to your situation, you should be closer to establishing a cooperative, progressive work group.

As you progress through this chapter, think of individuals in your department and assess what you have observed about each one to the evaluation material presented throughout this chapter. Keep in mind your team's mission and objectives and what you perceive to be key potential obstacles to developing a strong team so that the material herein becomes realistic, effective, and more practical in your own situation.

CONDUCTING A TEAM ANALYSIS

Great teams consist of great players. To build a team, you must first analyze the relative strengths and weaknesses of individual players, both current and prospective. This section discusses methods of analyzing strengths and weaknesses of individual members and developing a system to assess the potential, performance, and contribution of each one. To begin with, you will need a leader's notebook. In this one, make entries about your evaluation of each member (try to be as objective as possible). Use the six basic sources described in the following subsections to compile your analysis.

Performance Evaluations

Performance reviews and documentation include the evaluations completed by your management predecessor. Remember that under the best of conditions performance evaluation is a subjective exercise; personal bias on the part of your predecessor might have entered into the equation. While reviewing individual employee files, make copious notes about perceived strengths and weaknesses and the employee's development needs. Note in particular any comments on the employee's ability to work with others and his or her contribution to the team effort. Try to gauge employee attitude and interpersonal skills.

Firsthand Observation

Write down your firsthand observation of each employee's progress. If your **new** employees are former peers, you already may have opinions about their performance level and ability to work as part of a team. Remember that this logbook is a compilation of your own subjective notes; it is not a legal document or anything that **can be used against you** in any manner, so be forthright in your note taking.

Credible Secondhand Information

As mentioned in earlier chapters, upon assuming your responsibilities as department manager, interview each employee regarding their goals and objectives, aspirations, and opinions on how to improve performance on an individual and departmental basis. Only ask questions that relate specifically to your particular department's activity, current team orientation, and established group processes. These answers can be most telling in terms of individual attitude toward team cohesion and group contribution.

Selected Interviewing/Selection Data

Seek out any useful information uncovered during the actual hiring process for applicants screened by you or by your predecessor. In most healthcare organizations, the human resource department has copies of interview score sheets or similar data that will give insight into the employee's attitude, people skills, and team orientation. Most of these professionals are very skilled at extrapolating data obtained in the selection process which can be quite helpful in assessing potential team orientation. In conducting applicant interviews, additionally, always ask about teamwork experience and how highly group interaction is valued.

Probation Performance Records

Some healthcare institutions designate the initial 3 months of employment as a probation period. This means that a new employee's performance is closely monitored and assessed for a period of the first 90 days in a given job. More often than not, copious notes are taken by the reviewing manager and other individuals in the chain of command. Probation notes are a great means of determining the employees' team orientation, individual strengths and weaknesses, and a wealth of other information essential to determining potential value to the work group.

Other Resources

Several other resources can help evaluate individual performance relative to team contribution. Certainly the job description, combined with your perception of the individual's ability to meet the performance standards delineated in the job description, is important. It is vital to examine how each employee performs the job, conducts herself or himself in the workplace, and acts as a source of information and supportive player.

Furthermore, it is vital to examine individual potential and promotability in terms of technical acumen. (Technical acumen would include how much a compensation specialist knows about the hospital's employee benefit program or how much a pharmacist knows about decongestants.) A simple standard to apply in this case is determining what the individual's present level of expertise is, and how vigorously he or she pursues new technical knowledge and business acumen.

Finally, perhaps the most telling resource of determining caliber of team orientation is simply to observe collective departmental behavior. The following 5 questions can go a long way toward determining an individual's team potential:

1. Toward whom do people seem to gravitate in times of crisis?
2. Which individuals seem to be most willing to share technical knowledge?
3. Which individuals become actively involved in orienting new members to them?
4. Which individuals seem to work consistently in isolation?
5. Which individuals seem to provide leadership to the team by virtue of example, communication, and inspiration?

The answer to these questions, combined with the information from all of the sources mentioned throughout this section can go far in giving you a general perspective of your team **leaders and followers**. They can also give you an idea of who the more reluctant team players might be and whom you might target for specific individual team involvement.

QUALITIES OF A STRONG TEAM PLAYER

As you conduct your team analysis, several characteristics and work-related behaviors should be identified and quantified. This section will review several of these qualities and provide guidelines for identifying them, and a profile will be presented that you can incorporate into your efforts for the selection of new staff members.

The composite in Figure 7–1 provides some insight into what qualities a strong healthcare team member might possess. The model can serve as a building block in formulating a team blueprint.

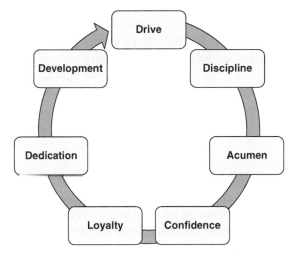

FIGURE 7–1. Traits of a strong team member.

Drive

Each team member must have a certain amount of drive to attain individual and group goals. He or she does not need to be **jump-started** every morning or at the beginning of each shift. The drive toward performing strongly, learning and growing every day, being a motivator for others purely by example, expending energy, and applying on-the-job initiative all characterize a stellar team player.

Discipline

Good teams are disciplined. They steadily make exact determinations and seek all facts necessary to making a decision. They get the job done correctly the first time and do not cause little problems that can add up to big problems. Good teams know intrinsically what has to be done and how to do it; that is, they set their own objectives and determine a course of action for achieving those objectives with excellence. Their sense of discipline is self-perpetuating throughout the entire department.

Acumen

One thing that makes the healthcare field so unique is the combination of many technical talents synergized into one greater whole. Every employee on the payroll of a healthcare organization has a certain amount of technical acumen and expertise that they bring to the job every day. Whether that expertise lies in conducting a **good** laboratory assay, filling a prescription correctly, or cleaning a patient's room quickly and efficiently, strong team members bring their unique, essential ability to the workplace every day. Never taking a **know-it-all** attitude, a strong team player looks at every day as an opportunity to learn something new.

Confidence

Every team member should feel self-assured about his or her technical ability and the resilience to perform under changing and critical circumstances. A strong player usually radiates confidence about departmental goals and everyday work activities. Both customers/patients and fellow workers pick up on this attitude and therefore feel comforted by this individual's presence. They have the conviction that the job will get done and that when the going gets tough—an everyday occurrence in health care—the job will still get done.

Loyalty

Team loyalty is critical in health care, and each player's loyalty cannot be selective or sporadic in its application. The first loyalty, of course, is to the healthcare institution and its mission of providing care to its patient community. The second loyalty is to the department manager/team leader and is demonstrated by following set objectives, providing feedback, and accomplishing team goals. The third loyalty is to the work group, to act as a positive participant who contributes to group goals. Finally, the individual maintains a dedication to always escalating their individual strong performance and progressive development on the job.

Dedication

Strong team members emanate dedication to a common goal of providing stellar health care to all customers/patients. They are equally dedicated to all team goals, departmental objectives, and one another in providing help, guidance, and technical assistance. They are passionate in their allegiance to the healthcare profession and equally dedicated to providing whatever support is needed to meet the healthcare mandate of premium service delivery.

Development

Each team member should desire to grow and develop on the job. This development, however, expands itself beyond the parameters of basic technical growth. Strong healthcare team members seek to learn more about the healthcare business and to understand the changing dimensions of the business. They know how to interpret the impact of change in the social environment and in their communities, and they understand how these changes may affect their particular duties and the institution's mission.

An often-overlooked aspect of team member development is interpersonal skills. A strong team member seeks to learn more about individual personalities and the proclivities of fellow team members and what their professional preferences and personal likes and dislikes might be relative to performance. This focus on development of interpersonal skills contributes significantly to an ever-expanding knowledge base from which the employee can grow, prosper, and continuously improve the quantity and quality of the work contribution.

ANALYZING WORK PERSONALITY

In industrial psychology and management philosophy circles, much discussion surrounds a concept known as work personality. The work personality of a healthcare employee is basically defined as **how** a job is performed, as opposed to **what** is done. As public scrutiny and customer/patient perception healthcare delivery become more intense and more keenly focused, the attributes of work personality relative to healthcare employees become increasingly more important.

In conducting a team analysis, you may find it useful to identify the attributes of work personality present in your team, as well as to study their effect on team performance. This effort can help deal with employees who go to extremes in performing their jobs, thus creating performance problems for the team. For example, an employee performing his or her job in an extreme manner is a strong performer who becomes a **workaholic** and pressures coworkers to work to his or her unrealistic standard. Several strategies and systems aid in analyzing work personality of healthcare employees. One of the most widely used work personality profile systems is the Quantitative-Communological Organizational

Profile System (the Quan-Com System) used by more than 150 hospitals. The Quan-Com System has been endorsed by several major healthcare accreditation organizations. This system may be useful for studying your team orientation and work behavior. Using this in turn can help you more accurately determine the team development needs of your staff and the individual tendencies and liabilities of your team members.

The basic elements of this system are attitude orientation, people skills, managerial aptitude, and team orientation. As they relate to the analysis of potential interactions and performance within your department, once again it is valuable to write in your notebook behavior and actions that might indicate a prospective member's propensity for constructive or nonconstructive behavior in any of the four areas, which are described in the following sections and subsections.

Attitude Orientation

First, review each employee relative to a series of attitude orientation characteristics. These characteristics include adaptability, accountability, perseverance, and work ethic.

Adaptability

Individuals lacking on-the-job adaptability are inflexible, reluctant to learn new methods or adapt to new ideas, and have difficulty relating to varied personalities. On the other hand, one who is too adaptable is said to be wishy-washy, unwilling to take a stand, or changes with any minor fluctuation in the work environment.

Individuals who demonstrate adaptability in good balance can adjust well to new methods and ideas with excellent practical results. They also are flexible in dealing with a wide range of people, reacting proactively and positively to change, and developing not only a Plan A, but also a Plan B in accomplishing set objectives. In essence, these individuals are versatile and can accommodate change positively, function well in crisis, and set new goals readily as circumstances dictate. This behavior is illustrated on the adaptability bell curve shown in Figure 7–2. You can draw similar bell curves for other attitude orientation factors to chart **pluses** and **minuses**. Write the initials of team members who represent points along the curve relative to their behavior.

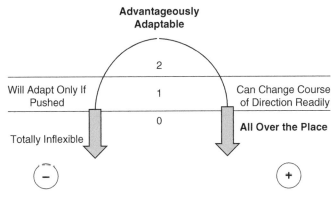

FIGURE 7–2.   Adaptability.

Accountability

Another attitude orientation factor is accountability. Individuals who demonstrate this characteristic are able to make a stand and stay with their objective without wavering in their position. These individuals take command appropriately in all business situations, and they are enterprising, direct, and persuasive in their business dealings.

Individuals whose behavior falls along the **minus** range of the curve (see Figure 7–3) usually will not take a stand on major issues and are overlooked by managers. At the other **plus** extreme are those who are too aggressive or pushy and may be characterized as obnoxious, overbearing, or offensive. They alienate fellow team members and over time become isolated or, worse, create the unneeded difficult situations.

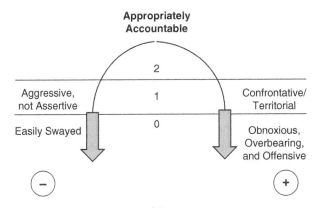

FIGURE 7–3.   Accountability.

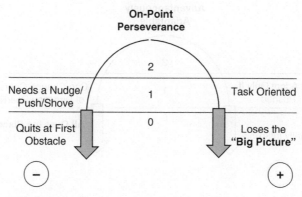

FIGURE 7–4.   Perseverance.

Perseverance

The third attitude orientation factor is perseverance. Perseverant workers are consistently persistent and tenacious in accomplishing a goal (**stick-to-itiveness**). They forge ahead tirelessly to a successful end despite situational obstacles. These players tenaciously assist fellow team members in the pursuit of group objectives (Figure 7–4).

Individuals who lack perseverance will quit at the first detour and usually bring someone down with them. That is to say, their malaise and resistance toward accomplishing a goal can act as a negative contagion and affect the morale and motivation of other team members.

Too much perseverance leads to tunnel vision; that is, these players are task oriented at the expense of being mission oriented (**can't find the forest through the trees** or **lose the mission at the expense of the effort**).

Work Ethic

Work ethic is encompassed in some of the work personality factors already discussed. For example, the work ethic is fueled by drive and dedication on the part of healthcare workers who stick to a job until it is done and have a basic industriousness (Figure 7–5). Team members lacking this quality eventually will be identified by fellow workers as unreliable and excluded from the team equation. On the other hand, too much of a work ethic can define a workaholic, an unfortunately common figure in the high-stress healthcare arena.

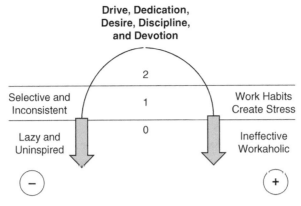

FIGURE 7–5.   Work ethic.

People Skills

The second category of the Quan-Com System for examining work personality is people skills. These skills fall into three general areas: communication, perceptiveness, and presence and bearing.

Communication

You may find it useful to analyze the communication abilities of all individuals in your department, including the ability to deliver a message clearly and with comprehension. Similarly, you may want to analyze members' various energy levels (Figure 7–6). High-energy individuals are

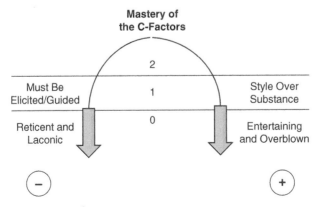

FIGURE 7–6.   Communication.

enthusiastic, enthralled by their work, convey a sense of electricity in their encouragement to others, and are eager to take on all new responsibilities and new challenges.

Perceptiveness

Perceptiveness relates to the insight individuals possess in dealing with others. Perceptive workers understand the people equation as it relates to the healthcare team process. Those lacking in this quality focus on people only after a problem surfaces, as they tend to be oblivious to the people aspect (Figure 7–7). At the other extreme are **overly perceptive** individuals, who focus on personalities and interpersonal problems at the expense of programs, processes, products, and objectives.

Presence and Bearing

In weighing the concept of presence and bearing, simply ask yourself "What would I think of this individual if he or she was the first person I came in contact with upon coming to the hospital?" The answer will tell you what customers/patients and fellow workers perceive about this particular team member (Figure 7–8). Presence and bearing—overall demeanor—denote the positive or negative impression created in a business situation.

Managerial Aptitude

Creativity is simply defined for our purposes as the ability to come up with new ideas and creative solutions to problems. Part of this aptitude is

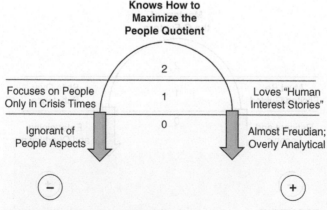

FIGURE 7–7.   Perceptiveness.

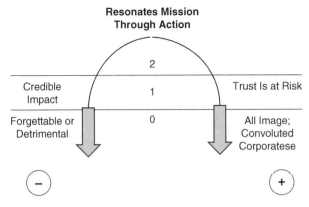

FIGURE 7–8.   Presence and Bearing.

the ability to delegate responsibly to expedite service delivery and effectiveness of action. By exercising independent judgment, a worker makes decisions autonomously when necessary. Finally, managerial aptitude relies on the ability to construct plans and make preparations for significant action.

Managerial aptitude might not be critically important in some areas. For example, if most members of your department are classified as nonexempts, nonskilled, or hourly employees, managerial aptitude might not be an essential quality. It is, however, essential to have team members who are relatively creative, can make plans, and use their own common sense in executing action. A preliminary analysis of each individual team member will disclose his or her strategies for enhancing these abilities and managing individuals who demonstrate varying strengths and weaknesses in these work personality areas.

Team Orientation

Our final category of work personality analysis addresses the very issue of this chapter—team orientation. Strong teams cooperate, relate well to peers, are loyal to the organization, and have the requisite technical expertise.

Cooperation is the ability to work as part of a team and to interact cohesively with other team members (Figure 7–9). Truly cooperative individuals can coordinate activities with others, act as leaders within the team structure, and value team participation and group activity.

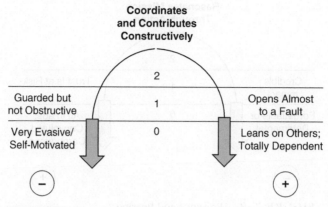

FIGURE 7–9.   Cooperation.

Individuals with no sense of cooperation act autonomously and in isolation from the team. They may become subversive and self-motivated to the point of destroying team morale and group interaction. At the other extreme are healthcare workers who are so team oriented that their individual contribution is suspect, who often refer to **we** as opposed to **I** when discussing business situations and accomplishments.

Employee relations, an important component to team orientation, might also be described as peer relations or the ability to work within a group when the term refers to individuals in a nonsupervisory capacity (Figure 7–10). Individuals who relate well to peers enjoy a productive and progressive work relationship with other members of the team.

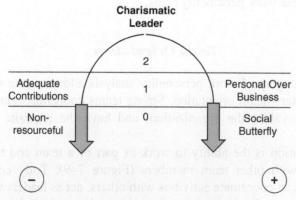

FIGURE 7–10.   Employee-peer relations.

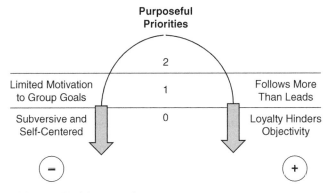

FIGURE 7–11.   Loyalty.

Loyalty (Figure 7–11) and technical expertise (Figure 7–12) have already been discussed, but remember that extremes in either characteristic should be avoided. For example, you would not want a subversive or disloyal member or one who lacked sufficient technical expertise. Nor would you want a player whose loyalty was misplaced or a pure technician who was unable to share information with a team spirit.

PERFORMING WORK PERSONALITY ANALYSIS

Using the 4 main elements of the Quan-Com System (attitude orientation, people skills, managerial aptitude, and team orientation), analyze the potential strengths and weaknesses of all team members relative to their

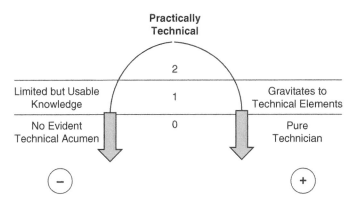

FIGURE 7–12.   Technical expertise.

potential to contribute to group goals. You can perform this important inventory using the figures contained in this section. Like other areas of management, your preliminary judgment will be somewhat subjective and certainly not a quantitative exercise. Next, do a preliminary inventory of each individual's preferences, tendencies, and liabilities. This can be done by dedicating a page in your notebook to each team member and dividing each page into three columns that represent the individual:

1. Peferences for work assignments and teammates with whom they enjoy working
2. Positive aspects of work personality
3. Negative aspects of work personality and teammates with whom they dislike working

Having accomplished this, you are now ready to look at setting up a plan for team accomplishment, which includes determining what type of team you presently have and, more important, what type of team you want to have. By now, you already know that you have an assortment of talent and a variety of personalities and team orientations among current staff (the rule rather than the exception). The next section will explore what kind of teams you can construct and methods of reinforcing team orientation based on individual strengths and talents.

ESTABLISHING TEAM ORIENTATION

As a new healthcare manager, chances are you are inheriting a ready-made team. No doubt your department has already been selected and has worked together under the leadership of your predecessor. To create your own team orientation and build (or rebuild) a team, first examine the current team. Even if you are the exception and are in the process of forming a new team, the following guidelines can help establish the standards you wish to incorporate into your team-building and team-orientation efforts. First look at what makes a strong, winning team.

Hallmarks of a Successful Team

These eight qualities mark a winning team:

1. Motivation to excel
2. Credibility and respect

3. Progressiveness in taking action
4. Inspiration and the will to be successful
5. Talent, expertise, and ability
6. Allegiance to the group
7. Achievement orientation
8. Spirit and positive outlook

Motivation

A team that attains its stated mission successfully and effectively is well motivated. Motivation can come from a variety of sources, the first of which should be the department manager. Motivation can be positive, where encouragement and progressive action are emphasized, or negative, where less-than-satisfactory consequences due to failure to meet team objectives are emphasized.

Motivation also must come from the work group itself. Individuals must inspire one another to greater performance and support the efforts of all team members. Also, each team member must be self-motivated (as evidenced by drive, which was discussed earlier).

Credibility and Respect

Because it is known for **getting the job done**, a strong team earns credibility and commands the respect of customers/patients and other departments. Strong teams have a wide base of technical knowledge and can readily provide whatever level of assistance is needed. Such teams are self-perpetuating, attracting and retaining other strong members.

Progressiveness

A progressive team grows continuously and develops expertise in an ongoing effort to enhance quality outcomes. Teams become progressive by valuing individual contribution, constantly attaining new technical knowledge, and experimenting with and implementing new methods of practices. Conversely, a regressive team loses ground, fails to participate positively in organizational activities, and its members are labeled **losers** throughout the organization.

Inspiration

Great teams are inspired by their will to win. Their individual members are success driven, and their leaders reinforce the importance of succeeding. This combination is the basis for inspiration. So that teams remain inspired, clear goals must be established, outcomes must be defined, and methods of attaining success should be delineated by the leader, with the participation of all members.

Talent

Without the expert talent and ability needed to achieve desired ends, a team is doomed to failure. Talent encompasses technical knowledge, performance ability relative to current healthcare mandates, and awareness of business objectives within the context of those mandates.

Achievement

All teams want to achieve on an individual, group, and organizational level. In making their contribution, team members must be challenged to become the best they can be. Therefore, you must foster educational development, training opportunities, open communication, and goal attainment for each staff member.

Spirit

As with leadership spirit, team spirit can be described as supportive, positive, result-oriented, or winning. These descriptives relate not only to the perceptions others have of the team, but—perhaps more important—to the team's perception of itself. **Losing** teams are characterized as whiners, dysfunctional, or negative.

CONDUCTING A TEAM PROTOTYPE ANALYSIS

Teams are formed for a number of reasons, and they either succeed or fail for a number of reasons. This section will help you determine what kind of team you need and will provide clues as to probability of success. The following subsections will guide you in taking an inventory of your current team so as to determine what type of team and team atmosphere you need to create.

Getting the Job Done

Some teams are formed simply to accomplish a particular task. This team is described as a matrix management group and might exist only over the short term. In examining your department, determine whether certain individuals should be paired (or grouped) together for a specific function or completion of a specific task.

Failing to Recognize Teamship

Poorly designated teams do not even realize that they are in fact work groups. Several individuals who work together on a constant basis may not see themselves as **doing teamwork**. A solution might be to officially designate a subgroup as a **team**, for example, if several individuals in your accounting department handle accounts receivable, you might designate them as the **AR team**. This helps individuals form an identification, and it clearly delineates for the team the lines of support. It also increases their morale and sense of affiliation, while enhancing their communication flow—both within the new team and throughout the department.

Being Numerically Oriented

Every team should be numerically oriented. For example, an athletic team measures its successes by the team's won-lost record; a non-profit theatre group quantifies its success by how much endowment money it receives and the number of performances it does in a given year. Teams must have a measurable goal (eg, repeating no more than a certain number of laboratory tests due to lost patient charts). Establish measurable numerical goals (**significant numbers**) using percentage, time, numbers, and fiscal indicators.

Some numerically oriented teams are **bottom liners**, that is, oriented to success strictly as measured by numbers. For such groups (eg, an accounting department, which naturally is driven by numbers), set numerical goals to attain. You might prefer to use score sheets or some other device to chart progress over time. Use time-sequenced progress charts as comparison guides and, depending on your management style, share them at department meetings or post them in a prominent place in the department. This will serve as a constant reward/reminder for the group.

Defining Team Objectives

Some teams are thrown together basically because each member has a lot of talent. However, members' commitment is shaky because they have not been shown how to work together. Establishing a sense of cohesiveness through clarity of objectives is the intent of the continuous quality improvement (CQI) process. If faced with this problem, you might consider holding a group meeting for the purpose of defining objectives for the team, specifying how each talent can contribute to the group process, and allowing the group an opportunity to answer the question, "How can we achieve collectively at the highest possible level?"

Another team may have medium talent but high commitment, which may be a preferred combination to the one above. Individuals with high commitment can sharpen their talent by working together and supporting each other's efforts to grow and develop. The cohesion demonstrated by this type of team can be used to increase interaction, define responsibilities, and identify ways to synergize talent and commitment effectively.

Using the Real Superstars on Your Team

Many teams have charismatic players who can have a positive or negative effect on the entire team. These individuals are usually very outspoken, typically have been on the team a long time, and have a certain degree of credibility with other team members. Seek out their allegiance at the beginning of your management tenure. If they affect the team negatively by virtue of their poor performance, document their performance, meet with them to put them on notice, and, if necessary, recommend termination. Provide positive performers with extra attention. Ask them how the team might get better and how members who might not be **up to par** can be supported. Enlist their support in developing the team and identifying areas in which the team can improve and grow.

In addition to star players, a team has steady players and low achievers. Use your superstars as role models and sources of positive motivation. Encourage their participation in group meetings. The steady players (probably most of the department) should be dealt with individually to learn their perceptions on how to increase performance, how to enhance goal attainment, and how they might contribute more strongly to the group. Underachievers are generally disinterested in their work and have no innate drive to improve on their activities. Document their work during performance evaluations, and, if necessary, recommend termination.

Establishing a Mentor System

Usually, a work group has a mixture of **rookies**, individuals new to the department (and perhaps the organization), and **veterans**, individuals who have been on board and working in the field a long time. This team mix can be used to great advantage if you implement a mentor system; that is, assign newer members to work with the more seasoned staff on a regular basis. Use your positively motivated veterans to help orient new employees, train rookies, and provide support for the entire department.

Using Veterans Effectively

Some work groups include individuals who have worked for the organization a long time and are experts in their technical field. These expert veterans can be a tremendous asset if most of them are motivated positively. Draw on this considerable resource by asking "Given that you've been in this business for quite a while, what can we do to become even better?" On the other hand, teams whose veteran players appear burned out or complacent may need to have the fires rekindled. Try arriving at individual goals or discussing with the personnel department ways to boost the performance evaluation process so that tenure and experience can be rewarded in line with performance.

Recognizing Opportunity

Although a rare occasion, you might inherit a team of rookies. That is, the majority of players have not worked in the field for long, are new to the organization, or both. A visionary manager craves this opportunity to work with a clean slate. If this is the case, use the suggestions in Chapter 9 regarding developing and educating staff. Remember, however, that in this scenario, a disproportionate amount of time will be required for training and development.

Capitalizing on Familiarity

If your department players already know each other, have worked together for a while, and therefore know each other's strengths and weaknesses, use this familiarity as part of your orientation efforts. Begin your team-building efforts by asking individuals how they can improve, whom they consider to be the stronger players, and what weaknesses the team may face as a group. Do not focus on individual weaknesses because employees may fear a **witch hunt**. Remember to take input from team members as subjective perceptions to supplement your own perceptions, not as an exclusive or definitive source of information.

On the other hand, teams that have never worked together and thus are unfamiliar with individual dynamics again provide the opportunity for you to work with a clean slate. Your main strategy should be to establish policies and operational procedures. Additionally, much effort should be directed toward educating your staff concerning your own objectives and desired expectations and toward developing individual goals for all members.

Capitalizing on Past Successes

If the majority of individuals on your staff worked in departments that have been successful, you have a great advantage. Primarily, these individuals will contribute to the motivation, spirit, and inspiration necessary for a winning team. Usually these individuals are steady performers who know how to win. Use them as role models, sources for suggestions, and proponents of positive contribution.

On the flip side, individuals who have worked in groups that have not been successful or that have been depicted as losers may have difficulty responding to positive motivation. If this is the case, you must impart three messages to the team. First, encourage them to focus primarily on the present and the future. Second, ask their opinion as to why past contributions were so unsuccessful and what their perceptions are on improvement. Finally, use performance assessment and observation to determine whether the cause for poor achievement lies with the individual (or certain individuals) or with some other dynamic (eg, outdated policy, budget cutback, or suspension of training program).

Benefiting from a Family Orientation

Family-oriented team members are socially cohesive and genuinely enjoy interaction with one another on a personal level. This type of team has both advantages and disadvantages. An advantage is that people will naturally support each other and work cohesively. On the other hand, certain individuals may be considered "the black sheep" of the family. Try to determine whether the family dynamic leads to cohesion and consonance, or dissension and dissonance based on performance or personality issues. Maintain objectivity—do not play the matriarch or patriarch role. Neither should you arbitrate disputes. Attempt conflict resolution by keeping the emphasis on performance, and apply the strategies in the next subsection to underscore your role as a leader, not as a parent.

Allowing Independence

Some teams are predominated by experts with outstanding technical acumen in their specialty area. These teams often operate on the principle of autonomy; they are self-motivated, self-directed, and function more or less independently. Do not try enforcing a group perspective onto such a team; rather, take advantage of each member's expertise and meet with team occasionally (not regularly) to share ideas. Keep the conversation tied closely to technical issues and ways in which technical data can be shared. Do not worry about socializing within this group or enforcement of strident interpersonal standards. Doing so can have a counterreaction which can further distance these key contributors.

Maintaining Status Quo

Certain teams are very happy with the status quo; that is, they do not crave opportunities to improve their performance. Like the jaded veterans described earlier, these team members may need a new dose of motivation. Try to ascertain what might reengage these individuals. Following are five suggestions for reinstilling motivation for the status quo team:

1. Explore new areas for creative activity.
2. Identify the performance dynamics of each individual member (**what makes him or her tick**).
3. Establish new goals for each individual.
4. Establish new goals for the entire department.
5. Implement a reward system, for example, conferring **employee-of-the-month** status that includes some unexpected but welcome rewards such as an afternoon or shift off from work beyond normal vacation time.

Work closely with both your supervisor and the human resource department to see positive ways to shake up the status quo team. Usually there is an inordinate amount of dormant talent that simply needs a wake-up call.

Identifying the "Collective We" Team

Certain teams are so group oriented that they see themselves as a **collective we** rather than a collection of individuals united in a common goal. These teams are considered to be **galvanized** (using popular jargon), meaning that they function as a unit and often will move only as fast as the slowest member or work only as hard as the laziest member. Sit down with each member to discuss individual goals and objectives, keeping the conversation focused on **individual** contribution. Discourage discussion of group activity, but without denigrating the importance of working cohesively. Clarify your position that the standard for excellence will be the expectations set by the best worker in the group.

Identifying the Leader-Oriented Team

A **leader-oriented** team, the easiest type for a new manager to inherit, will closely monitor the behavior and actions of the new leader and apply those standards and outcome observations to their own work. Therefore, strong, effective leadership (as described in Chapter 2) is the best strategy for generating progress on a leader-oriented team. Remember that in this case—as in the case of all types of teams—your actions, words, and plans will be closely scrutinized and evaluated by all members of the team. So if you are fair and forthright in your actions and exhibit behavior that helps group progress, you are off to a good start.

REINFORCING TEAM ORIENTATION

Remember, establishing team orientation is not an exact science; numerous strategies are available to help you constantly reinforce a team concept within your department. These strategies are drawn from the checklist of team qualities in Figure 7–13.

The first strategy is to **establish common objectives** for the team. Let all team members know the objectives of the department and the main mission of the department in your estimation as well as in the eyes of the organization. Remember that management involves asking the right questions. Question your staff about their perceptions as to the main objectives of the department and the common goals toward which individuals should be striving as member of the team.

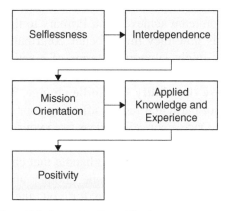

FIGURE 7–13. Essential elements of an effective team.

Feel free to **share your perceptions** with all members of the team. Let them know what your opinion is on various organizational issues without appearing disloyal or lacking in allegiance to organizational objectives. This will encourage individuals on your team to share their perception and their perspectives on organizational initiatives, as well as their insight on how to achieve departmental objectives that will contribute to the good of the organization. Achievement is centered on the individual and enhanced by group action. Thus, the sharing of perspectives and perceptions is vital to establishing team orientation, and the lines of communication is vital to a strong team.

Remember that diversity of talent characterizes a successful team. **Recognize individual talents** and ask for suggestions on how their individual talent might be applied to the team. In the attitude surveys conducted by the authors, a number of employees indicate that they have many suggestions but have not been asked by their manager to share them. The best source for learning how to synergize individual talent into group contribution is the individual department member.

Keep Feedback Lines Open

Encourage two-way feedback between members and yourself. Ask their opinions on your management style and on the way that the department is progressing toward stated goals. Listening skills and perception skills are important elements of decision making, as well as contributing to the group process. Again, use the questions in this text as a model for asking the right questions on team achievement. Primary to this set of questions is asking individuals how they might better contribute to the group, as well as whom they might support in terms of creating a greater team effort.

Good teams **have the ability to handle change**. Try to identify any changing dynamics or particular factors affecting your department as pro-actively as possible. Once again, elicit ideas from your staff on what areas of change might be apparent relative to their particular jobs and, more important, how they can best prepare to handle that change successfully. Encourage all members to motivate one another and to support one another through transitions. As is true for you, the team's ability to bounce back from adversity is a hallmark of success. As a healthcare manager, you may have to reassign individuals occasionally to help team members who require extra assistance. Rely on veterans and stronger players to provide this assistance, which will not only help achieve objectives but also increase team allegiance and individual motivation.

Provide as many opportunities as possible for your team to **grow, learn**, and **develop**. Present as many in-service exercises as possible, and utilize the expertise within your department to present new ideas to the group. One strategy in this area is to have **show-and-tell** sessions, where team members explain to each other new principles, strategies, and methods of accomplishing technology-based ends.

Hold meetings at least once a quarter to **establish new goals** for the department. Review past goals and accomplishments, seek explanations for why goals were either achieved or not achieved, and seek input from the group concerning their perceptions as why goals were (or were not) achieved and objectives met. Make this a group process to ensure credibility as well as maximum input and opportunities for shared knowledge.

Never discount the degree of scrutiny or underestimate the power of perception on the part of a team observing its leader. You must consistently provide **strong leadership**, using the guidelines offered in this chapter. As discussed in Chapter 4, exemplary leadership is fortified by executing decisions and actions that put the best interest of the team and the organization at the forefront. Provide clear direction on a daily basis, both to the individuals within the group and to the group itself. Take the time to renew your perspective, as well as replenish staff spirit, by conducting quarterly progress review, inviting suggestions, and encouraging participation.

Always **make sure that your team has the resources needed** to get the job done. The key word in this sentence is **need**, and the vital necessities for performance should be provided by the organization with your assistance as the healthcare manager. Remember that as circumstances change, the need for additional resources might change. Therefore, keep up to date on the needs and desires of your team, as well as your subgroup.

Finally, keep in mind that **team orientation is a balancing act**. The balance between freedom and control, individual and group performance, and personal motivation and organizational spirit can be maintained mostly by clear vision, open communication, and progressive action. As a healthcare manager, recognize the importance of progressively analyzing individual strengths, team orientation, and utilizing commonsense strategies to encourage team achievement and garner group performance.

Any attempt at introducing the practical precepts of ethics and value-driven action (VDA) programs into a healthcare setting must be anchored in realistic expectations, practical packaging, and a direct intent at producing meaningful outcomes and results. A specific needs analysis must be conducted at the outset of the program to ascertain not only what will work, but perhaps more importantly, what will not work—or even be considered tenable—by members of the healthcare organization. This latter point is extremely important, as the healthcare professional has been deluged with a variety of organizational development programs whose banality is insulting, irrelevant, and faddish. The outcome of these programs is one of two reactions:

- "So what? We still have problems, the hospital is still empty, and I'm gonna get laid off!"
- "They (read: leadership) spent good money that could have been better spent on our salaries/needed supplies/saving jobs/taking care of patients."

In any semblance, these outcomes destroy the trust that is required between leadership and staff in any successful healthcare organization.

The VDA organizational development effort must not have a trendy name or any features which can be construed as phony, inauthentic, or faddish. The CQI **Quality Craze** among healthcare organizations left a multitude of healthcare professionals with a justifiable antipathy for any **trendy**, insincere attempts at organizational renewal. A realistic outlook must be considered by leadership, with an emphasis on a need for commitment by a majority of organizational members to at least **give the program a chance**, as opposed to the unrealistic desire to have a total consensus by the entirety of the organization. There will always be dissension, notably on the part of the **nonplayers** who are self-absorbed, self-professed **victims** of anything and everything that the organization undertakes in a positive, honest attempt to better the workplace. If the VDA program is to be successful, it will stress:

Outcomes over opinions

Product not process

Results over remorse or retribution over past events

Individual accountability and performance contributions to the organization

Meaningful intents and objectives

A different approach from total quality management and other failures of the **process/psycho-babble** era

To accomplish a real-world, practical organizational development process, the PACT System delineated in Chapter 2 of this book must be put into action in a team-oriented application.

Pride

A major motivational factor in any organization, health care or otherwise, is the genuine investment in the organization through action and performance which is inspired by true pride in the organization. A seemingly eclectic roster of organizations such as the United States Marine Corps, the Xerox Corporation, and the Girl Scouts all have withstood various travails and organizational strife—and indeed, developed and advanced through time and change—due to the feeling by their members that each member was, simply put, **part of the best**.

Popular components of daily argot such as "Send for The Marines", "make a Xerox copy," and "Girl Scout Cookies" did not enter the lexicon accidentally.

Accountability

The worst statements that can be uttered in a healthcare workplace within hearing distance of a customer/patient are:

That's not my job.

We don't do that here.

I don't know.

All these excuses convey clearly to the listener that the individual uttering these banalities does not care about patient health or customer service, but moreover, confirms the worst suspicions harbored by the customer/patient community, as delineated in the initial paragraphs of this article.

The VDA program must stress individual accountability and positive action which reflects credit on the organization and a clear responsibility to upholding its mission and objectives.

Commitment

The commitment to the principal four constituent groups of a healthcare organization is mandatory to the continued success of the organization and the individual.

In the proper order, these four constituencies must be the everyday targets of optimum performance by all members of the organization:

1. The customer/patient, who ultimately drives the organization and controls its destiny, and who displays their commitment to the healthcare organization by virtue of their patronage as demonstrated by emergency room visits, physician support, and participation in bake sales

2. The organization, which displays its commitment to an employee by providing employment which represents the opportunity of using all of one's talents in the pursuit of providing healthcare services to those in need of healing

3. The team/department, which coordinates and synthesizes individual talents into an expert, competent, able group which can fluidly provide service in an efficient and effective manner

4. The individual, whose commitment to their own maximum professional and personal development is facilitated by the daily rendering of top effort to all endeavors

Trust

Perhaps one of the few absolute certainties in industrial psychology is the erosion of trust and the absolute inability to regain trust after it has been forsaken in any semblance. Employees, physicians, specialized staff, and volunteers can all have the same reaction to a real—or even perceived abridgement of trust: if you **burned** me once, you'll likely do it again! Indeed, even the manner in which new VDA programs are introduced must be authentic, **straight-shooting**, and clear if any hope of building— or in some cases, regaining—trust is to be realized.

OPERATIONALIZING THE VDA PROGRAM

Once a commitment has been made to developing and implementing a value-driven organizational development effort, the innovation and installation of several strategies should be initiated. Eight fundamental programs can be customized, introduced, and incorporated into the fabric of the healthcare organization at a relatively low cost and with minimal consultant or other **outside** effort. This latter point is vital, as the perception that any organizational development program has been developed by a consultant for the benefit of the consultant's wallet rather than the progress of the organization's 4 main constituents is the precursor of failure for the entire program's implementation.

Eight programs that fit into the organizational development efforts at most healthcare organizations are:

> **House rules:** A listing of customer/patient relation strategies which can be detailed and printed in on a laminated card can be a good reminder for guest relation standards and moreover, serve as valid, criterion-based performance factors. At many hospitals in New Jersey, these standards became the **flip-side of each employee's name badge** and were linked to their **Whatever It Takes** customer service program. Outstanding performance was rewarded with a meritorious bonus—a needed auspice of any **people development** program in health care.
>
> **TimeLines:** The future plans of the organization, as well as a general review of its organizational performance over a yearly period, can be easily published as a TimeLine depiction of organizational performance and shared with all employees, physicians, and volunteers. The VA Medical System in Hawaii, consisting of four separate facilities on four different islands, found that the publication of TimeLine reviews and TimeLine strategic plans in an annual report for the coming year was a terrific conveyance of getting commitment and understanding from all members of the four facilities.

Targeted selection system: As described in our chapter and resource, the creation of organizational standards for targeted selection can quantify performance standards at the essential **how we do it** level. Using the interviewing questions and cues in Chapter 4 of this book is a great start to implementing a structured selection system.

Criterion-based, values-driven performance evaluation systems: A major motivational tool, for both the marginal performer and the **superstar** employee, is the annual performance evaluation, such as the system apparent in the previous chapter. However, when the performance evaluation is merely a **checklist** review of the existing job description, it becomes virtually impossible to distinguish the great performer from the goldbricker. At Jane Phillips Medical Center in Bartlesville, Oklahoma, a performance evaluation which measures how the individual performed relative to job specifications, assesses the CARE or PACT Factors of attitude orientation, people skills, and team orientation, and recognizes contributions made beyond the set job description has been a key element in the renewal of this important, urban nonprofit facility. The practical resource in our book is a starting point for you in this important initiative.

Volunteer education: Consider for a minute how many volunteers are present every day in your healthcare facility. Whether you measure by numbers or percentages, the likelihood that they become instrumental in the perception formation of your customers/patients is very high. Holy Cross Medical Center in Los Angeles found that inclusion of the volunteers in every educational forum ensured that the volunteers were on **the same page** as the paid staff members, and moreover, that a clear understanding was established regarding essential **house rules** and performance standards.

CRI surveys: Attitude surveys have been used to the point of tedium and inefficacy over the past 10 years. It is a fair assumption to conclude that their impact has become negligible due to overuse and the confluence of media and organizational input which leads the survey respondent to **guess** the right answer.

The Change Readiness Index (CRI) featured in this book is a scorecard system in which a respondent rates the organization in the categories of customer/patient service, organizational reaction and readiness to change, and overall organizational dynamics such as communication and morale. The VA Medical Center in Phoenix, Arizona used the CRI to assess the right strategy and approach for not only the commencement of a new leadership team, but additionally, for strategy formulation in every new venture undertaken in their immense growth.

Execugrams: There is no such thing as **overcommunication** in a healthcare organizational setting. The use of periodic **execugrams** which are correspondence from the CEO of a facility to all working staff members and volunteers is an easily implemented management tool. At the Mercy Health System in Oklahoma, these messages were coded in green and contained information ranging from a favorable bond rating to news of the opening of a new clinic. The use of an alternate color other than white for the execugram ensures that document **stands out** beyond the tonnage of usual missives delivered on white paper stock.

Executive Commitment: The chief executive of every healthcare facility and their second tier of leadership—that is, all the executives who report directly to the CEO—should undertake various new tasks with a renewed commitment to their own accountability. Many failing healthcare organizations like to expound on their commitment to employees, quality care, and all the other platitudinal mantras. Three questions can usually be asked to determine if commitment exists at the executive level or the stated commitment to value-driven leadership is polemic driven:

1. When was the last time the executive walked completely through, around, and down all corridors and crannies of the facility?

2. When was the last time the executive asked a random employee for any ideas on how to improve the facility at large or merely the quality of staff work life?

3. When was the last time the executive asked introspectively, was I honest, direct, and hardworking in all I did on this day?

If the answer to any of these questions is anything besides, **today**, the outlook for success of the value-driven action program is nil. In the final analysis, a commitment to decency, a sense of pride regarding the organization's mission, a deep-seated sense of leadership accountability, and a demonstrable ability to trust all involved in the caring process is the ultimate value-driven action program. With it, the healthcare facility meets the charter of caring for those in need in the best traditions of American health care; without it, it's just another place where sick people go because **they have no choice.**

The most important choice is the decision made by the healthcare leader at every level to make value-driven action a daily, constant requisite of selfless service, not a fad or a **sometime thing**. The good news is that most of us in health care have a desire to lead a life worthy of our professional calling; the bad news is that we often get bogged down in nuances which cause disorientation from our precious mission. Renewal is easy if it is truly desired: hopefully some of these ideas will give you a place to start.

SUMMARY

Just as individuals are different and work under differing circumstances, each team is unique. Therefore, no one solution serves to establish team orientation. The worst mistake a new healthcare manager can make is to expect that a group of individuals with diverse talents and differing perspectives will work cohesively and consistently. The team process takes time, so communication must be ongoing. Common goals must be stated and adjusted with changing circumstance, and positive motivation must be provided in healthy and abundant doses.

The saving grace of establishing a team is that most healthcare workers are well motivated to provide stellar service to the customer/patient. Use this as your vanguard in getting immediate results in establishing a strong, cohesive team.

PRACTICAL RESOURCE—CHAPTER VII:
General Project Plan (GPP) Guidesheet

This resource is a guide for the healthcare/physician leader to plan project objectives and scope with their staff, incorporating all of the significant tenets of this chapter.

Project Name:

Project Leaders:

Rationale/Mission (Why?):

1.

2.

3.

4.

5.

Goals/Objectives (What?):

1.

2.

3.

4.

5.

Process, Plan & Program (How?):

1.

2.

3.

4.

5.

Timeline & Timing (When?):

1.

2.

3.

4.

5.

Human Capital & Consumers (Who?):

1.

2.

3.

4.

5.

Significant Indicators - including percentages that represent performance, fiscal indicators, time quotients, and working numbers (How Much?):

1.

2.

3.

4.

5.

Locations and Physical Resources (Where?):

1.

2.

3.

4.

5.

Engagement Keys/Call to Action (Why Should/Do I Care?):

-

-

-

-

-

-

-

CHAPTER EIGHT

Encouraging Creativity and Innovation

Doing more with less is a frequently echoed healthcare mandate that demands strong creative contributions from each team member. Although everyone on your team is probably creative, methods to stimulate creativity and a progression of creative management techniques help maximize this essential resource. To be progressive and to achieve its goals and objectives, a healthcare organization must tap the creativity of all workers throughout its ranks but unfortunately, in many healthcare environments, creative ability goes untapped. For example, some organizations are highly structured and do not encourage or reward creativity. Other organizations encourage creativity but do not progressively reward creative contribution. For a healthcare organization to survive and thrive, it is essential that all members attempt to make creative contributions that generate positive results and further the organization's goal of high-quality and affordable patient care.

As a newly appointed healthcare manager, you have a prime opportunity to foster a creative environment within your department and to set precedent with the plans you implement and the policies you incorporate into your management approach. Creativity not only helps in organizational achievement, it also acts as a positive catalyst within a department, as it improves morale and fosters a sense of participatory allegiance.

The opportunity to be creative inspires participation from all members of the staff and demonstrates to them that what they bring to the effort is valued and vital to the organization's success. Creativity is essential to the growth and development of all members of the organization. To grow and develop on the job, your staff must stretch its wings and venture into new areas and explore new methods of achieving results. As mentioned, creativity is a primary healthcare mandate. With customer/patient placing new demands on providers and needing services that heretofore were either nonexistent or unavailable, it is critical for each member of the healthcare organization to offer ideas that might meet these consumer demands.

This chapter will explore the prerequisites for creating an environment, examine the fundamentals required to encourage creativity throughout your department, and, most importantly, provide you with specific strategies for boosting creativity and garnering new ideas and approaches from your staff. These objectives will be accomplished with a view toward how you as a new manager can apply these strategies to your own personal development while using them to institute new programs. After reviewing these strategies, you will be able to build a creative environment in which to exercise your own management responsibilities.

ESTABLISHING A CREATIVE WORK ENVIRONMENT

To develop a creative team process, the work environment must be conducive to breeding new ideas and new approaches on the part of workers. Furthermore, your team members must know that their creative thought will be valued and rewarded, so that they do not feel afraid or intimidated to present creative solutions. This of course, is easier said than done, for reasons that will come to light in the following section and subsections. As this chapter progresses, you will be presented with group and individual strategies that will help facilitate the creative process.

The team creative process begins with identifying individuals among your superstar and steady employees that will be helpful in establishing the proper climate for creativity. With this objective in mind, review the following specific list of your more positive, likely creative contributors:

- The true superstar
- The new team member
- The previously disenchanted individual
- The technical expert (or **techie**)
- The **untapped steady**

Once again, although running the risk of stereotyping, you are simply categorizing personality types who will help you establish a creative environment. These are the likely depositors into your creative idea bank, and they strongly and fully support your efforts. Many of these individuals have been hungry for the chance to provide creative input, and your new presence represents for them an opportunity to liberate their ideas. These individuals will be like a strong thoroughbred who merely must be guided and directed toward the finish line as you run for the roses.

The True Superstar

True superstars are the positive leaders in your department who possess most of the technical knowledge and consistently demonstrate stellar professional ability. Their very presence and approach to the daily undertaking of their work responsibilities indicate that superstars are employees who would **run through the wall** for the organization. They will become your demonstrable role models for the work group and will always be ready and willing to present new, creative input that will lead to positive action.

Draw on these individuals heavily in the creative process. Ask for their opinions and input first in your work discussions and have them summarize their objectives and intentions at the end of the meeting. This will also underscore the type of performer you value on your staff. Furthermore, make certain that you clue these people in, without playing favorites, prior to any creative meetings. For example, upon a chance encounter with a superstar the day before a creative input meeting, give him or her some specific objectives to think about and ask that he or she be ready to share input at the upcoming meeting. Superstars provide a stellar contribution to your staff and hence deserve the reward of special consideration. Again without showing favoritism, show respect for their ideas and give them the maximum opportunity to contribute—which they richly deserve.

The New Staff Member

The new staff member can also be prime contribution to the creative process. For example, new members recently arrived from other institutions may have a wealth of ideas on new applications for their work activities. They also may have several ideas of what worked or did not work at their previous institution. Hence, they might have some new angles that can benefit your staff and help spark forward thinking in your creative meetings. You also might have new department members from other parts of the organization. They also will have new ideas and approaches and a sense for what did or did not work in their previous department.

Once again, tap these sources for their creative input. Their immediate participation will help make them part of the team right away, and they and the **veteran** team members will get to know one another at once. Hopefully, they will get off on the right foot in establishing their work role within the department and will be positively drawn to your other strong players.

The Previously Disenchanted Individual

A less obvious but likely creative contributor is the previously disenchanted individual. In many cases, new managers take on responsibility for a department that is in trouble. Put frankly, you may have gotten your job because your predecessor had a large hand in the department's poor track record. In many scenarios, new healthcare managers are replacements for predecessors who were totally ineffective, too authoritarian, or simply were not sound communicators. Individuals who worked under such leadership may have been strong performers but became disenchanted and disengaged from the staff performance process. They fundamentally did their own thing, without regard to departmental progress or team contribution. They likely were strong performers and well-motivated individuals prior to your predecessor's arrival.

Once again, you have a prime opportunity to use the creative process to achieve overall greater staff performance. By allowing these disenchanted players the opportunity to contribute and provide their input, you are recognizing their abilities and demonstrating clearly your esteem for their performance. In many cases, they will respond by returning to their previous high-level motivation. Remember to also examine the dynamics of their job descriptions and daily work responsibilities. One technique in this regard is to spend a day with each individual in your department at the outset of your management tenure. Constantly ask questions to learn as much as possible not only about the work role but also about the individual. This establishes an excellent precedent for dialogue and allows you to spur their creative and innovative thinking right from the outset.

Workers with a negative attitude for any number of other legitimate reasons might also fall into the category of the disenchanted. For example, their job may have been restructured for good reasons; the lines of report may have changed; or they may be suffering inordinate stress created by workplace circumstances that may now be smoothing out. In each case once you have identified the person as disenchanted, delve not so much into the circumstances of what created their outlook, but apply your efforts toward positive action.

For an individual who has a negative attitude, identify what created the negative attitude. If it is something that is job related, consider restructuring or reorienting the job role and the basic job description. If it is something that does not pertain to work but rather is generated by the individual's personal life, you might want to get an assist from your personnel department or an employee assistance program. If the negative attitude was specifically pertinent to the actions of your predecessor, simply ask this individual for a chance to prove yourself as a manager, thereby enlisting his or her support and participation. If the individual fails to respond to any of these actions, you no longer have a potentially supportive team member—you have a nonplayer performance problem.

The Technical Expert

As discussed throughout this book, most of your staff are technically proficient or **techies**. For these individuals, their work interest is founded in the technical application of their jobs. They have a strident affection for these technical angles, even though they sometimes may appear to live in their own little world. This work is defined by the parameters of their technical aptitude and the responsibilities that specifically utilize their technical expertise. A strong healthcare manger plays to the strengths of these individuals while ensuring that they continually have opportunities to participate fully in the work of the team.

The Untapped Steady (Figures 8–1 and 8–2)

Additionally, **techies** can also fall into the category of the **untapped steady**, an individual who endeavors to put in a good day's work for a fair day's wage but could be enticed to give a little more if approached appropriately. Like techies, untapped steadies are interested in the organization, but heretofore have never been specifically challenged to make creative contributions. Involve them in the group process, specifically charge them with idea innovation directives, and, regardless of category, make the process as engaging and enjoyable as possible.

Advocate – A positive voice in a process who shares a keen, progressive belief in the value of the action.	Exploit – Although the word has a negative connotation when applied to the mass media, as applied to management lexicon, exploit means to publicly utilize and recognize positive action and exemplary results.
During times of change, it is virtually impossible to over-communicate to staff members, especially steadies who act as advocates during the change process. Leaders who can first identify the likely advocates among their steadies and then activate their dedicated participation.	Satisfaction, recognition, and affiliation are key motivational agents that act as catalysts to the advocates during times of change.

FIGURE 8–1.   Steadies as innovation advocates.

STIMULATING INNOVATION INPUT

It is essential to use some techniques immediately upon entering the management ranks to establish a creative environment. This section will discuss several techniques you can incorporate into your style to make the creative process part of your everyday positive work actions.

Playing to Individual Strengths

To begin with, remember to play to individual strengths. That is, encourage an individual who has a strong technical proficiency to come up with

Level 5: Borderline Superstar

Level 4: Technical Superstar

Level 3: Steady for Life

Level 2: Gravitator/Escalator

Level 1: Borderline Non-Player

FIGURE 8–2.   The five types of Steadies.

technical ideas and newer specialty innovations that might bear on the entire department. Widen your scope as you do this; for example, ask a radiology technician how he or she might improve laboratory performance outcomes utilizing existing resources and providing stronger service. Then, using that person's own activities as a base, ask what might be done to encourage stronger intradepartmental cohesion—that is, how others in the department can better support this efforts of other in the department.

This process can be started, as mentioned, by utilizing a **spend-a-day-with program**. Upon assuming your management responsibilities, try to spend a day with each individual on your staff. Try to learn the specific objectives of each department member and the specific dimensions of his or her work role. This activity will also help you in the creative process, as you will get ideas on potentially reorganizing the department, restructuring certain jobs, and utilizing all the resources in your department more fully.

In undertaking this endeavor, present each individual with a brainstorming notebook. Ask each to record any ideas that answer the following questions:

- What can I do to make a stronger contribution?
- What resources would I ideally like to have to get my job done?
- What new and different approaches have I heard about or read about relative to my technical area?
- What new and different approaches have I heard about that might assist us in becoming a better department or better organization?
- What **wild and crazy** ideas have I considered and think they might actually work and generate positive results?

With this notebook approach, you are formalizing the creative process. Each individual will see clearly that idea generation will not be your exclusive domain but a team effort in which everyone's participation is encouraged and valued. To follow up on this technique, try to hold meetings at least monthly, but certainly quarterly to review all new ideas generated and allow everyone the opportunity to offer their ideas and present any suggestions that might bring about positive action.

Asking Questions and Gathering Ideas

As discussed repeatedly throughout this book, it is vital to ask questions throughout the creative process. Numerous questions have been provided throughout the text that you can use in a variety of management situations.

Always ask questions on both an individual and a group basis. This not only allows you to get answers that are pertinent and valuable to your own management activity, it also encourages all members of your staff to ask questions. As posed by a popular media advertising campaign several years ago, great companies always ask "What if...?"—in a similar vein, the biggest question you can ask in the creativity process is "What would happen if...?" Always present ideas, and try to get the up side and down side of incorporating any new ideas or new programs into your daily activities. After all, if you do not ask the question, you will never get the answer, and you might be missing something that could be valuable to your departmental activities.

Many organizations take asking questions a step further by holding what are commonly called **blue-sky meetings**. In blue-sky meetings, individuals are charged with looking at the short-term and long-term perspectives of their department, and while considering their department's future, they are asked to ascertain specifically what mission and objectives the department should be pursuing. In following this strategy, they try to innovate plans that accommodate these new suggestions. If you use innovation notebooks and give each individual in your department an idea notebook, you have a ready-made resource to use in these meetings. You can supplement this effort by simply asking, "If you had a magic wand, what would you make it do—besides making the hospital disappear or crating a perfect world?" This is yet another way of generating new ideas and allowing people to expand thinking in a free-flowing manner.

Encourage individuals to consider all sources in their idea generation. This would extend not only to other departments within your organization but to any ideas that they might have heard or read about in the media. It can also include ideas from organizations that they are involved with, aside from their healthcare employer. For example, they might belong to a community, civic, or religious organization that utilized a successful management or customer satisfaction system.

Most times, customers/patients are also neighbors of the organization's employees. Therefore, individuals in your department probably have access to a vast repository of ideas on how to improve service and, certainly, on common perceptions of the institution held in the community. Some of your staff members might have heard comments about your healthcare facility and specifically about your department as compared with other provider organizations and departments. This can also be a tremendous source of ideas and potential new applications. Finally, their previous job experience and the input they hear from peers within the organization might be yet another untapped resource in idea generation, which can be collected in their idea notebooks and presented in your meetings.

Most of the individuals in your department attend some sort of education and development programs. They could be programs presented by a technical organization, a civic organization, or in-service education within your institution. In all of these activities, your staff hears the perceptions and ideas of other individuals. Once again, they should bring significant input back to your idea generation meetings and record in their idea books specific comments that might be helpful. For example, a dietitian might attend a national association meeting and come back with ideas on a food program used by a hospital in another state.

Individuals attend retreats and workshops that might have very little to do with their technical areas, as these functions engender their participation by virtue of their membership in community organizations. Once again, some useful ideas could be generated. Furthermore, in some healthcare organizations, managers go on retreats to discuss basic issues and receive the benefits of professional education. This is yet another source for new creative ideas, as are weekly meetings when conducted as illustrated in Figure 8-3.

Regardless of what idea sources are used, it is incumbent upon you as a manager to identify the value of acknowledging and recording potentially useful ideas. No idea is a poor one—it is simply that some ideas have more merit and potential application to the workplace than others. Therefore, it is important to identify the importance of considering all sources in idea generation, to encourage all members of your staff to

Win of the Week	Learning Point of the Week	Play of the Week	Idea of the Week
Guest of the Week	Group Objective of the Week	Organization Objective of the Week	Player of the Week

FIGURE 8–3. The **Weekly Meeting 8**.

present these ideas, and to reward individuals who contribute new ideas through recognition and other merit systems.

Utilizing the I-Formula

To provide you with an even more concrete framework for bringing imagination and ingenuity into your workplace, this section presents the I-formula, which was devised by the authors for use by military officers in the late 1970s and has since been adapted and utilized successfully by thousands of healthcare managers. It is a simple approach to inspiring innovation in the workplace and making imagination and creativity an everyday part of the healthcare workplace. This section will review all elements of the I-formula, explain the importance of each element, and utilize case study examples of a healthcare manager's application of the formula in dispatching his or her own responsibilities, as well as a case analysis of healthcare manager who used the formula for his or her staff.

The formula is structured in four phases: need, design, action, and establishment. Each phase is further divided into six subphases, for a total of 24 I-components.

Phase I—Identifying the Need

A creative process begins with a need or an opportunity to improve the status quo (see Figure 8-4A). The need phase begins with an inspiration.

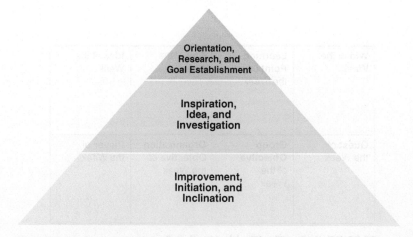

FIGURE 8-4A. The need phase.

Inspiration

Inspiration is the inspired motivation to create a new process or a new application. Without proper inspiration, the creative process cannot take place; with inspiration, a clear goal is defined and individuals can begin to contribute pragmatically to the creative process. Although the inspiration for addressing a need should be defined and communicated by you as manager, it can be suggested by any member of your staff or any other participant in the action area, such as a supervisor, colleague, or customer/patient.

To illustrate the I-formula, we will follow the progressive utilization of this strategy by two healthcare managers, Jenna Chang and Shane Flanagan, who hold very different positions in two healthcare organizations. Shane, a human resources director at a small-town clinic, has been told by his boss that turnover is an increasing problem among the clinic's staff of 60 members. The inspiration, provided by the clinic director, is to identify the root of turnover and to stop its negative effects.

Jenna is the chief operating officer (COO) of a long-term rehabilitation facility. She has decided to come up with a new guest relations program that will accurately collect the perceptions of discharged customers/patients.

Idea

The second segment of the need phase, the **idea**, is a potential solution, or a set of solutions, that might meet the need specified in the inspiration. Once again, the idea should be generated by members of your staff and ratified and clarified by you, the manager. For Shane Flanagan, the human resources director, some potential solutions include engaging an outside consultant to conduct a survey or a set of exit interviews. For Jenna Chang, the ideas range from customer/patient surveys, demographic analysis, and a wide range of other solutions.

Investigation

The third segment of the need phase is **investigation**, which is extremely important at this point, when all viable options are considered to be based on potential effectiveness, maximum use of available resources, and overall potential to produce a high-quality final product. The investigation should be conducted by the most expert members of the staff, under the leadership of the department manager; it should utilize all the talent available.

The investigation must be accurate, comprehensive, and realistic in scope. Otherwise, the entire process can be a failure.

After considering a wide variety of options, Shane Flanagan has decided to conduct exit interviews. He feels that use of questionnaires utilized by individual managers will be cost-efficient and user-friendly and will generate the data necessary to ascertain the root of the turnover problem in his organization. Jenna Chang has decided that her segment of the healthcare industry relies on the personal touch. Therefore, she will utilize follow-up call system, which (as will be shown) is also cost-efficient, user-friendly, and seems to be the best bet to achieving the desired results.

Improvement

The fourth segment of the need phase is perhaps the most important. If no **improvement** can be measured or directly recognized by implementing a new process, the entire process is a waste of valuable time and effort on the part of the healthcare staff. Although individuals like to be creative and to arrive at new and different solutions, a distinct improvement must be made. To draw an analogy, the best pharmaceutical companies are those who not only perform research but develop new drugs. To carry this 1 step further, the difference between research and development is that development yields new and better products.

Initiation

The fifth segment of the need phase is initiation. At this point, individuals will present their ideas to other appropriate members of the organization, members of their staff, peers, and superiors. In this context, the word **initiation** has dual applications. First, effort will be made to initiate the participation of all members of the staff and the organization so that they can contribute their thoughts and offer suggestions on how to improve the process at hand. Second, initiation refers to a period set aside for orientation of all appropriate members of the organization to the problem at hand, to at least provide them with knowledge and offer **membership** into the creative process.

Shane Flanagan has scheduled a 15-minute meeting with all members of the hospital's executive team in the interest of getting their ideas. He will also make some preliminary comments as to how they might participate in benefits they might gain from the process.

Jenna Chang, on the other hand, has decided to talk informally to all members of the long-term rehabilitation facility staff individually so that she can customize her presentation and ask specific questions to each member as appropriate to the process. Because she has five managers reporting to her, she will make sure that each member of the team has a discrete opportunity to participate in the process and to discuss perceptions with their leader. Both managers are new to this process, as Shane was previously a staff recruiter, and Jenna was a nurse team leader and both recognize that communication is the key not only to creativity, but to performance.

Inclination

The final segment of the need phase is **inclination**, the sum of personal preferences for action that will spell out the initial plan of action. For example, Flanagan has decided to use a set of six questions he has drawn from various human resource textbooks that can be used in exit interviews. Beatrice's inclination is to experiment with some survey questions herself, and make some personal calls to previously discharged residents in the hope that these questions can be fine-tuned for use by other members of the organization.

Phase II—Designing the Action Plan

The second phase of the I-formula, the design phase, begins with innovation and invention, as depicted in Figure 8-4B. The attempt now is to formalize

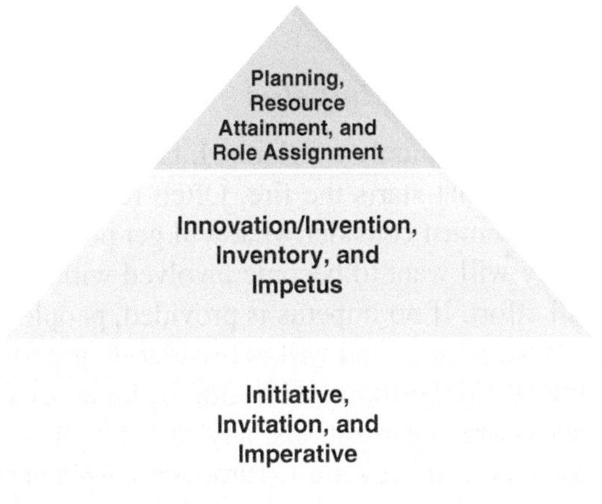

Planning,
Resource
Attainment, and
Role Assignment

Innovation/Invention,
Inventory, and
Impetus

Initiative,
Invitation, and
Imperative

FIGURE 8–4B. The design phase.

plans and to design a specific action plan for accomplishing the goal, which is to arrive at a new and creative process that meets an organizational need.

Innovation/Invention

Innovation refers to the utilization of existing resources to come up with a new process; invention mandates using unavailable (or nonexistent) resources to create (**invent**) a new process or product. A reality of health care is that an innovator is preferred over an inventor. The reasons for this are simple. With resources shrinking and available revenue in a state of constant decline, no healthcare provider truly has all of the resources desired. Most, however, have all of the resources **needed**. Therefore, an innovative style is preferred to an inventive style, as the innovator will have infinitely more opportunities to accomplish something.

Inventory

Tightly aligned with innovation/invention is inventory. **Inventory** refers to taking stock of all existing resources at hand, considering all players involved, and incorporating this inventory into the plan design.

Both case study individuals have decided on innovation over invention. Flanagan realizes that he simply needs a copier to make copies of the sets of questions he has for the exit interviews. Chang decides to utilize a process that just needs the participation of her staff and a clear understanding of the objectives.

Impetus

A most important, but commonly overlooked, factor in the design process is **impetus**—the spark that starts the fire. Often referred to in marketing terms as the **hook**, you must consider what will get potential stakeholders' attention so that they will want to become involved with your process and support the overall effort. If no impetus is provided, people will fail to see the importance of your actions and will not render their participation to its successful attainment. Furthermore, with time being an extremely limited commodity in healthcare organizations, any investment of time must be met with a guarantee of a strong return. Turnover has plagued all members of Shane Flanagan's organization; thus any solution that will alleviate this problem will be met with strong support and a positive outlook.

For Jenna Chang, however, the challenge is more formidable. She has several benefits that can be achieved by her efforts, including increased customer/patient satisfaction and an array of secondary data that will be gathered in her study and will help improve the overall quality of her facility and in turn the financial stability of her organization. However, she is using an element of intrigue in her efforts. Recognizing that people are naturally curious about **how they are doing**, she is using this human factor as part of her impetus strategy. She will simply ask members of her staff, "Wouldn't it be interesting to find out what our customers/patients really think about us?" Any motivated player on her team will answer this with a ready affirmative, and thus she will have both attention and positive support of all members of her staff.

Initiative

Initiative is the basic drive to see the design process through to its logical end and to take ownership of the new process. In both cases, the players are clearly in charge of the action and will generate all the forms necessary to complete the action, assigning responsibility as appropriate.

Invitation

Two factors are closely related to initiative. The first one is **invitation**, where people are invited to become involved in the process. Shane Flanagan will invite three key department leaders to participate in his turnover study and exit interview process initially. Jenna Chang will invite any two of her five direct reports to participate on a voluntary basis in the first round of customer-patient action calls.

Imperative

Invitation can also be supplemented with the **imperative**. In certain cases, it is very important to get the backing of your leader and superiors in a new creative process. In some cases, this might mean your soliciting the involvement of your CEO or other executive players. In most cases, you should seek to get the support of your immediate superior so that the mentoring process can be further solidified and you can get the necessary authority (**clout**) needed to make your new process happen.

Both case study individuals have garnered the participation and support of their senior executives in the process. In Shane Flanagan's case, the CEO has agreed to send a letter to all members of the staff explaining the turnover problem, delineating its deleterious effects on the entire organization, and detailing the general aspects of his plan. In Jenna Chang's case, the CEO has raised the topic of customer/patient opinions and perceptions. As can be seen, the participation of senior members in the process provides an imperative to all individuals to become interested in the process. Moreover, it clearly demonstrates that the organization is interested in the outcome of these projects, has deemed them to be important, and has set a very clear expectation that everyone will participate and contribute toward its success.

Phase III—Implementing the Action Plan

Upon completing the need and design phase you now move into the all-important action phase, as delineated in Figure 8-4C. If the first two phases have been followed strictly, and each segment has been met with a certain amount of ingenuity and productivity, the action should be productive.

Instruction

Now that your plan has been established and a need identified and addressed, you must instruct individuals on what their participation will be relative to the new action. Many healthcare managers fail to orient and instruct individuals on new processes. Accordingly, fear of the unknown

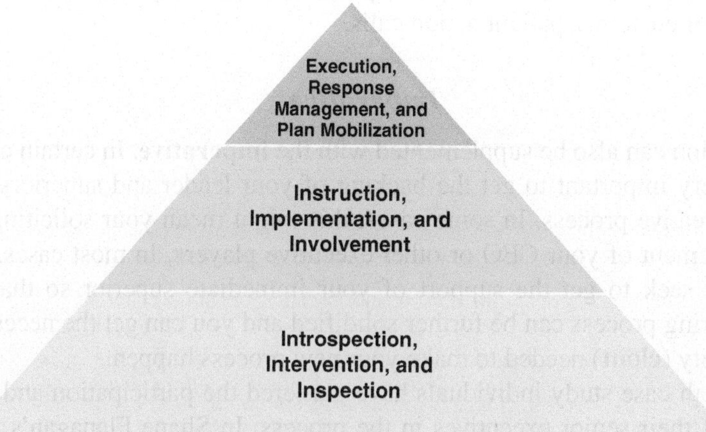

Execution,
Response
Management, and
Plan Mobilization

Instruction,
Implementation, and
Involvement

Introspection,
Intervention, and
Inspection

FIGURE 8–4C.   The action phase.

works in concert with fear of change in negating the creativity process. It is extremely important to educate all individuals on not only what is to be done, but how to do it.

For example, Shane Flanagan has set up meetings with his colleagues on the management staff who are going to use the exit interviews. He is instructing them not only in the purpose of the exit interviews, but also in the questions, and how to register responses appropriately. Furthermore, he will discuss possible outcomes and the possible perceptions (such as dissatisfaction with low wages, disgruntlement with superiors) that might be held by individuals leaving the organization.

Likewise, Jenna Chang is instructing all of her charges in how to get customer/patient feedback using her 10-part system. Because all of her staff members were interested in participating in the process, she is using this positive interest to get all of her managers involved. She is instructing them on when to make follow-up phone calls and what questioning procedure to use in the follow-up phone calls, and she is assigning a basic objective of 10 random calls per month to be conducted by each one of her managers.

Implementation

Initial implementations are referred to in the business world as **pilot projects** or **test runs**. The likelihood of achieving success across 100% of your organization on the first attempt at a new process is next to nil. However, many great ideas are lost due to this misguided expectation of first-run success. It is therefore essential to attempt to achieve success in a smaller area of the organization so that you can fine-tune your process and also engage the feedback of initial users who are meeting with success. Natural momentum can be built upon the success of few individuals using your process, which could elicit the interest of the majority of the rest of the organization.

Looking at the example of Shane Flanagan, we can see a prototypical example of this dynamic at work. Two of his colleagues, Maella Trujillo and Kyle Rowan, are department managers who have used the exit interviews. Following the use of the questions on a couple of occasions, both individuals have suggestions for rephrasing the questions to get a more comprehensive response. Lauren has suggested putting the questions in a format that allows the manager to fill in the responses as they are relayed by the outgoing employee. Furthermore, she has found it valuable to simply give the questions to a disgruntled employee, and allow him or her the opportunity to write down responses and mail them as convenient. These are very good suggestions that Flanagan can now incorporate into his process and utilize as he expands his efforts.

Involvement

Involvement rests on getting the full participation of all suitable parties throughout an organization who might benefit from your process. Once an implementation has been made and is fine-tuned and utilized successfully, involvement should be fairly natural progression in the process. Involvement can utilize not only members of the organization, but outside individuals such as colleagues at other healthcare organizations, professional contacts, or customers/patients.

Jenna Chang's team members have now made their follow-up calls over 3 months. Given the span of these 150 calls, she has collected a tremendous amount of information that will provide her with needed primary and secondary data about her organization and its effectiveness. However, to collate all the information, she is now seeking the involvement of a nursing school friend who has computer ability. Her friend, who works for a public organization, has graciously donated a couple of hours to Beatrice's nonprofit organization to show her a software package that will help her collate responses and present data in a logical fashion. Furthermore, she has secured the involvement of a member of the organization's board of directors who owns a printing business. This individual will print up the questionnaires and InfoCards, which can then be used by members of her staff and incorporated into the new computer scheme of tabulating and assessing information.

Introspection

It is important at this point for the manager to sit back and assess the action taken to date. This **introspection** is a period you can use for validating your creative process. Ask five important questions:

1. Is the process moving toward meeting the stated need?
2. What major lessons have been learned already in the process?
3. Am I using all of my resources successfully and efficiently?
4. What improvements can be made immediately on the process?
5. What will some of the long-range benefits of the process be?

Intervention

After answering these questions, you are now ready to accept intervention as needed. **Intervention** is any participation on your part to add creativity to the process and to develop the positive nature of the effort constantly.

Intervention need not be dramatic. For example, Shane Flanagan needs only to ensure the participation of other managers and not take any further personal action himself. However, Jenna Chang has a good opportunity to increase intervention in her efforts. First, upon introspection, she has determined that follow-up calls on her behalf as facility COO will be quite useful. For example, two particular previous customer patients were quite upset at the lack of consideration they felt they experienced upon calling the facility following their discharge. In such cases, Jenna has decided to follow up with a phone call herself, in which she identifies herself as the COO of the facility, states that she understands the problem, and pledges to try to provide some practical positive action. In doing so in these cases, she has alleviated the complaints and, more importantly, increased the satisfaction level of these previous customer patients by her progressive action.

Furthermore, Jenna has decided that the participation of the board of directors is key to the success of the program. This suggestion, fully supported by her boss (the CEO), entails having each member of the board make five calls a month to previous customer patients in the interest of determining their level of satisfaction with the facility and its services. The entire organization recognizes that the board's participation in this process will add another point of view to the process and is a very creative method of assuring the customer patients that the organization truly cares about their welfare and is vitally interested in constantly improving its efforts and services.

Inspection

The action phase concludes with an **inspection**. A comprehensive inspection should include answers to the following 10 pertinent questions:

1. On a grade of 1 to 5, with 5 being high, how would we rate our action at this point?
2. If the score is lower than 3, should we go back to the drawing board, starting with the need process?
3. If the score is higher than 3, how can we make it a solid 5?

4. What major organizational benefits are being realized by the process?
5. What additional resources might be needed to make the process even more fruitful?
6. Are our expectations being met realistically?
7. Is this new process contributing to the values and ideals of the organization in a progressive manner?
8. Should others be involved in the process?
9. Should other actions be taken to improve the process?
10. Given the best of all circumstances, how can we make this process part of the realistic day-to-day action of the facility?

If you are satisfied with your inspection checklist, you are ready to proceed to the final phase of the I-formula, the establishment of long-term change.

Phase IV—Establishing Long-Term Change

The objective of the establishment phase is to provide a sound answer to Question 10 of the preceding list by making the process an ongoing part of the organization's activity. Figure 8-4D provides an illustration of this pivotal phase of establishing long-term, positive change.

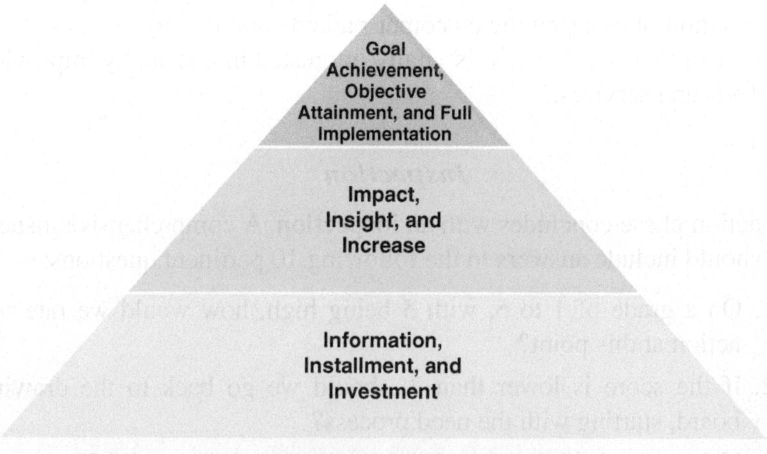

Goal Achievement, Objective Attainment, and Full Implementation

Impact, Insight, and Increase

Information, Installment, and Investment

FIGURE 8–4D. The establishment phase.

Impact

At this point you are measuring the impact the new process has had on the organization. Reviewing both case studies, Shane Flanagan has now been able to fine-tune his exit interview process to the point that all managers in his small hospital are utilizing the questions when an employee leaves the organization. Not only has this made the managers aware of the dilemma caused by turnover, it has sent a subtle signal to the employees that management is concerned about the turnover.

In Jenna Chang's case, customers/patients who are at the facility currently are aware that managers will be calling following their release and are naturally now looking at services more closely. Additionally, all members of the organization—particularly those reporting to Jenna's five managers—are keenly aware that their efforts are being closely evaluated. The impact of this action is twofold. First, individuals are taking more pride in what they are doing and are appreciative of the good feedback they are getting relative to their work efforts. Second, Jenna is aware of the fact that in the future, individuals will expect the opportunity to provide feedback upon their discharge.

Insight

Now that the new creative process has been established and utilized by appropriate members of the healthcare organization, insight and opinion should be collected from all users. For example, Jenna has asked all members of her team for suggestions on how to make the process better and in fact has used all the questions appearing in this section. As a result, she has gotten the new idea of providing InfoCards to all discharged customer patients. This includes giving individuals a questionnaire when they leave the facility, which augments the random phone calls.

Increase (Positive Gain)

Increase relates to any improved productivity evidenced or generated by the new process. The insight provided by Shane Flanagan's efforts is that employees are leaving the facility strictly because the benefits and wages do not compare favorably with the marketplace. Consequently, he has conducted a wage survey and has gotten the board of directors, with his supervisor's help, to approve a wage increase and a strengthening of comprehensive benefits package. A year from now, the turnover rate will have gone down, length of employment for the typical employee will have increased, and some other positive gains will have been generated by his efforts.

Information

Information is any kind of data or significant communication generated by new creative process. For Jenna Chang, a wealth of information has been provided relative to customer/patient concerns and, in fact, has helped set criteria for what constitutes a successful stay at her long-term facility. Through this information, another usage of the word **informed** comes into play. As word gets out through the grapevine in both organizations, both case players are enjoying certain benefits.

For Shane Flanagan, once word got out about the exit interviews and the benefits that are an effect of the exit interviews, top management of the organization authorized him to compile a set of questions that could be used during selection interviews, which would help identify and select individuals who could likely be retained. In Jenna's case, once all five of her managers used the customer/patient follow-up call system, all of the staff began to use the process—staff nurses, therapists, and even physicians affiliated with the facility.

Installation

These systems will now be **installed** into the organization, much in the manner that a new physical facility is incorporated into a larger structure. Installation occurs if the answer to each of the following 10 questions is a resounding yes:

1. Did the process meet a specific need?
2. Is the process user-friendly?
3. Did the process generate clear results?
4. Is the process viable?
5. Does the process underscore the ideals and values of the organization?
6. Does the process have a long-term benefit?
7. If the process has a short-term benefit, should we use it again?
8. Was customer-patient service improved by the process?
9. Were employee relations and motivation improved by the process?
10. Did the process help make the organization more productive and progressive?

For both Flanagan and Chang, the answer to all of these questions was yes. Although for educational purposes two cases were used that were very positive and idealistic in scope, both examples were taken from real-world situations and from the authors' experience over the past 2 years. The important thing is to understand the elements of the I-formula and to utilize its components effectively and efficiently as you try to bring creativity into your workplace.

OTHER CRITICAL FACTORS FOR LONG-TERM CHANGE

Three additional I-factors (Figure 8–5) should be considered in looking at the total spectrum of team creativity. First, recognize that **inertia**, the failure to move forward (ie, the state of remaining stagnant) unfortunately has taken hold in many healthcare organizations and departments. Hence, initially you may meet some resistance whenever you try anything creative. You must be the prime motivating factor, and by utilizing the tenets of this chapter you can gain the support of all appropriate parties to move things forward toward a progressive new goal. Two other factors, **importance** and **interest**, must also be underscored. Make sure that your new process is important and gets everyone interested in the process. By engaging the work interest of others, motivating their participation, and achieving some important new goals, you are bringing much-needed innovation and ingenuity to the healthcare workplace. Not only will this benefit you, it will serve the most important person in the healthcare organization—the customer/patient.

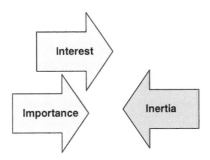

FIGURE 8–5.   Momentum Factors of The I-Formula.

SUMMARY

Creativity from all team members and resultant progression action are vital linchpins between potential and realized success. By optimizing the potential of all team members appropriately, garnering their creative input, and synergizing individual talents and contributions into a comprehensive and progressive work unit, you will ensure your organization that a substantial contribution will be generated by your staff. Furthermore, the customer-patient needs of your operating environment will be met by cohesive group of motivated, constantly developing professionals.

PRACTICAL RESOURCE—CHAPTER VIII:
I-Formula Leader's Checklist

This resource provides you with a quick preparation guide of planning a new project or program with a focus on innovation and creativity. It can be employed individually or with a group with equilibrant results.

Investigation

Imperatives:

Inspiration:

Impact factors:

Intrinsic assets:

Identification:

Imperatives

Needs assessment:

"Lay of the Land":

Realistic goals:

Desired outcomes:

Inspiration

Constituent dreams:

Traditions:

Institutional aspirations:

Recent history:

Crisis, change and chaos:

Impact Factors

Available resources:

"Looming presences":

Potential(s):

Possibilities:

Cures needed asap!!!:

Intrinsic Assets
Natural resources:
Play to strengths:
Address and/or negate weaknesses:

Identification
Immediate action:
Priorities:
Pressure points:

Plan of Action:
Artful participation:

Information
Input:
Ideas:
Instincts:
Insights:
Images:

Input
Formal:
Informal:
Documentation:
Visualization:
Comparisons:
Contrasts:

Ideas
Everyone counts:
Every idea counts:
Every moment is important:

Instincts

Value-driven:

"Gut Intelligence":

Immersion:

Not who you know; it's what you know about 'em!:

Insights

Over-communicate:

Listen proactively:

Right questions and the right time:

Images

3-5 element maxim:

General to specific:

"Boss" the message:

Action orientation:

Innovations

Implementations:

Improvements:

In-touch:

Intensity:

Influence:

Initiatives:

Implementations

Look for "naturals":

Logic:

Cogent:

"Picture this…":

Benefits x 4 (Patient, Organization, Team, and Individual):

Improvements

Positive images:

Creative confluences:

Critical Numbers - #'s, $, %, Time

In-Touch
Regular "check-ins":
E-mail:
Reports:

Intensity
Pressure points:
Acrimony, apathy, antipathy, and antagonism:
Solutions over problems:

Influence
Tell some progress stories:
Celebrate the wins:
Continuous communication and development:

Initiatives
Calibrated goals:
Progressive development:
Stay on message and…:
Keep building on the message!:

Call to Action
Essential elements:
3-5 rule:
User-friendly:
Active, action-oriented leadership:

CHAPTER NINE

Education and Development Strategies

EDUCATION AND DEVELOPMENT

Y ou can reap great returns from healthcare training and development efforts. It is often said that management is an art, very qualitative in scope, and greatly reliant on style. Others maintain that management is a science, technical and quantitative in scope and reliant on research and acquired expertise. Others maintain that management is a set of skills, which could be acquired through formal knowledge and then incorporated by individuals into their everyday activities. Still others maintain that management rests on pure magic, reliant on luck, gut feel, and basic instincts and is greatly dependent on the will of the managers to **do the right thing**, which in turn will provide its own rewards.

You have probably quickly realized that management and leadership are actually a combination of all of these dimensions, a true confluence of art, science, a set of skills, and magic, with the only constant being that you can never learn too many useful strategies. Training and development, when specifically applied to managers as a management development effort, can assist you in attaining competency in several basic areas. More to the point, it can help you in terms of developing your own abilities, with each experience providing an enriching and encouraging lesson in dealing with people and making yourself a better professional.

THE LEARNING CURVE

As Figure 9–1 indicates, you are currently on a management learning curve; over time, you will achieve a certain degree of competency. If you consider the figure and its charting of a manager's typical first year, it demonstrates how competency will increase each quarter as you acquire the skills charted in the graph.

Initially, you should try to master observation skills. Closely monitor the progress and performance of your staff, observe the actions of your peers, and study closely the styles and applications of the managers and leaders with whom you work. To the extent possible, listen to all experiences in all areas of expertise, and try to perceive each episode as a lesson. This will provide you with a basic frame of reference in management, as well as with some specific information needed to lead and mange the individuals on your staff. Observation will also help meld your relationships with peers and superiors.

The second phase of management is the trial and error. Typically this occurs in the second quarter, although certainly no time lines are considered absolute in every case. In the trial-and-error phase, try to establish some policy, make decisions, and operate as an agent of change within your sphere of responsibility. As you continue your education in this school of **"burn and learn,"** few things will work perfectly the first time, but you learn from your mistakes, get better all the time, and acquire some

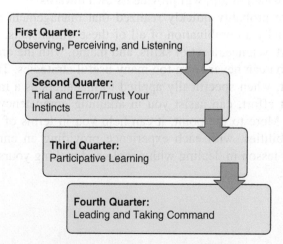

FIGURE 9–1. New healthcare leader's first year of learning.

expertise. The third phase, participative learning, takes into account the entire range of activities you will learn and grow from and apply practically to your business situation. At this point, you are probably acting as an instructor yourself in delivering information and providing instruction to your staff. Additionally, you are providing expertise to your peers and consultation to others who need your assistance. If you are keeping a logbook (which is highly recommended) and applying many of the techniques discussed throughout this book, this phase could be a very successful period, one that provides you with some much-needed positive reinforcement.

Mastery of the participative learning phase leads naturally to assuming a leadership role, the fourth phase of the curve. As a leader, you are on your own and have acquired a certain degree of competency—although you are still learning, which, hopefully, you will never stop doing. The worst risk you could incur is failure to stay current with new management techniques, innovative ways of dealing with people, and advancements that sharpen your technical acumen.

SOURCES OF LEARNING

As a new healthcare manager, you will receive information and education from a variety of sources. These sources include, but are not limited to, the following:

Peer input: The perspective provided by peers as well as their common experience in becoming healthcare managers can prove invaluable. Remember, all situations are not identical, and the circumstances under which they worked in their initial management phase might differ from yours. However, generally this could be a good source, as **these individuals have walked in your shoes**.

Personal experience: You own personal experience in health care which will be a valuable asset as you enter management. This experience is a source of information because you have acquired a certain degree of expertise and have certainly observed healthcare managers in action. Rely on your gut instincts as well as your own knowledge in terms of what does and does not work. Use this reference throughout your management career.

Related experience of others: The managerial experiences related by others in your organization (or by family or friends) can be very helpful.

Although the banking industry, for example, certainly differs from health care, certain aspects of people management share similarities. Once again, examine these experiences, ask questions, and try to gain knowledge from this important source.

Organization-generated education: Seminars, workshops, and other educational opportunities provided by an organization can be invaluable in establishing a reference point as a healthcare manager. Take advantage of any and all educational opportunities the organization provides, specifically those on management of healthcare business issues.

Journals and other reading: A whole body of healthcare management literature is available for your perusal and use. Try to select reading material that is practical in scope and provides information you can apply immediately. Ask peers and others in your organization whose opinions you respect, which periodicals they subscribe to and find most valuable. Most publications of the American College of Physician Executives and other professional leadership development organizations tend to be very practical in scope and provide valuable information that can be used immediately by newer and seasoned managers.

Formal education: Although many healthcare managers endeavor to attain a management degree, perhaps at the graduate level, it could be equally valuable simply to take a course that relates to a specific development need help in financial skills; certainly, your local community college or state university has a course on finance for the nonfinancial manager that can meet this development need. Do not feel compelled to acquire a new degree—simply pick the courses and seminars that are most applicable to your situation and will provide the most immediate feedback and value.

Project management: As always, keep a journal or logbook in which you will record any major projects you undertake or significant issues you must manage. Keep a chronological log of time and events, with an additional line displaying what you learned in each situation. This will provide you with your own textbook of management and give you a sterling reference for the next time you undertake a similar project or scope of responsibility.

Supervisors and mentors: Your supervisor can be a valuable source of information and a terrific educator if you are comfortable with the relationship and feel he or she has a certain amount of knowledge to offer. Furthermore, as will be discussed later in this chapter, the mentoring process is quite useful and has been adopted by many leading hospitals from an organizational perspective. Later in this chapter, appropriate individual strategies for mentoring will be delineated.

Staff input: The healthcare manager who discounts employees' ideas and input as being invaluable or unnecessary is doomed to failure. Although there are few absolutes in management, this certainly is one of them. Try to learn as much as possible from employee comments, viewpoints, and by simply observing them in their daily activities. If nothing else, you will learn how they are motivated, what they respond to, and what they deem as being negative within the workplace.

Outside networking: As mentioned in the preceding chapter, as you progress through your career in healthcare management, you will establish a network of contacts throughout the business. Whenever you meet a potential contact, exchange business cards. Use a Rolodex or small file cabinet to store the cards categorized by state, business type, or title (pharmaceuticals manager, personnel coordinator). This can be a useful source of knowledge and a **living library** of health-care management.

TYPES OF LEARNING

To promote your development as a manager, there are basic ways of learning new skills that you should always try to make time for: communication-based learning, formal learning, and experienced-based learning.

Communication-Based Learning

Communication-based learning consists of simple observation, formatted observation, question-and-answer sessions, and secondary or hidden discovery. Simple observation is the act of perceiving as much as possible just by experiencing situations and either mentally noting or writing in a journal or logbook any significant incidents and learning points from the experience. This opportunity is always available to you and gives you a realistic perspective of how to deal with problems and reach positive solutions.

Another form of communication-based learning is formatted observation, that is, the undertaking of a project with a colleague or staff member at the outset of which you specifically delineated what you want to learn from the experience. By establishing this **lesson plan**, you can undertake the experience with your colleague and achieve specific learning objectives from meeting. Ask yourself beforehand: "What can I learn from this meeting?" At the conclusion of the meeting, simply answer that question, and determine what you did in fact learn from the meeting and what possible educational benefit it might have for you. Strive to achieve two or three learning points from each type of communication-based learning.

Two other types of communication-based training directly support the entire idea of quality-focused healthcare delivery. Question-and-answer sessions are activities in which you ask point-specific questions about important issues. These sessions could be prearranged with a group of colleagues, or held in a one-on-one setting with an individual with a creditable range of expertise. Secondary (or hidden) discovery is any experience in such a manner that you learned a great deal. For example, this might have occurred at a meeting in which you saw someone manage a communication conflict or a customer/patient complaint and detail how they brought about a successful resolution. Once again, you need a notebook to record these observations and the benefit of your **hidden discovery**. Hidden discovery can extend to leadership style, management aptitude, or basic supervisory psychology. Once again, it is readily apparent and available for your use.

Formal Learning

Formal learning is at once the most obvious type of management education and, unfortunately, the least available. However, it is important and can delve into specific areas that might be of value to you in your role as a healthcare manager. Formal education can include reading and research, consisting of well-defined reading lists on management topics, such as the one contained in the bibliography at the end of this book or books recommended to you by your information and educational sources described earlier in this section.

Seminars and workshops are the second type of formal education. Be certain to attend those programs that are specific to your needs; avoid those that hint of trendy topics and very little meat. The way to determine this is to ask the instructor for a specific learning plan or simply discuss the content with the instructor using the material in this chapter's Practical Resource.

The third type of formal education is perhaps the most obvious—formal coursework. This can include a college course of other type of educational offering that will provide you with specific information over a defined period of time.

Most newly appointed healthcare managers immediately feel a need to pursue outside education in the form of a degree program. This is a natural reaction, due to their innate feeling that entry into the world of management mandates more credentialing. Actually, your promotion was premised on your potential and established performance as a healthcare professional as perceived by those executives who provided you with the management opportunity.

However, if you insist on undertaking a degree program at the outset of your managerial career, keep certain cautions in mind. The first problem is that because your time will be limited, you could be setting yourself up for failure. For one thing, achieving a balance between personal life and professional responsibilities can be tough enough without the additional burden of keeping up with a new school regimen. Your effectiveness might drop as your stress level rises. Furthermore, the natural benefit of education—absorbing new ideas and enjoying the positive interchange with fellow students—may be compromised by efforts merely to make it to class and put in your time.

Some who enter healthcare management without BA or BS degree— perhaps an individual who was an RN or a practitioner and did not complete 128 hours most institutions require for a degree—become preoccupied with immediate acquisition of a degree and may feel professionally insecure without it. Although finishing your degree work is important, it is secondary in your first year, which must be spent learning as much as you can about your staff, the supervisory process, and a myriad of techniques essential to becoming an effective healthcare manager. Once again, time is the most precious resource you'll need to manage during this period. Thus, the unnecessary intrusion of schoolwork into the equation will likely hurt your progress more than it will enhance it.

After your first year, it might be prudent to begin pursuing a new degree or competing outstanding coursework. As you consider your educational plans, the following guidelines might be helpful:

Pursue relevant courses. Whether you are considering a master's program or completion of undergraduate work, focus on courses directly related to your current responsibilities. This will give you maximum immediate return on your efforts while providing insight and instruction that can be applied at once to your workplace.

Avoid becoming a slave to the degree process. Attaining a new degree is a laudable accomplishment. It also takes an inordinate amount of time and energy, particularly if the program is a **tradi-tional** curriculum, which does not include weekend sessions or other more user-friendly opportunities, such as executive degree programs or night school. After reviewing course content, select programs that are most relevant to your job and development goals, not those that cater to instruction that can be applied at once to your workplace.

Seek out professionally oriented programs. Most progressive university programs are designed with the busy professional in mind. Such programs include weekend classes, credit for significant professional accomplishment already achieved, and faculty members who are in touch with the real world. This should be a major consideration in your decision-making process for the benefits are exposure to fellow professionals and a realistic and practical educational base.

Use moderation. At the outset of your new college work, take one or two courses that hold a specific value for your pursuits. This value may be defined, for example, by a course whose content may contain specific material relevant to your responsibilities or provide you with two or three immediately useful ideas for your management efforts. Either way, it may prove enjoyable to you. This approach—simply taking three or four courses that interest you and yield specific instruction in a key area, such as a graduate certificate program—may be more valuable than relentlessly completing an entire program and then wondering, "What did I get from that?" Remember, your time is limited, and your main qualifications for the current job and future opportunities are your past achievements and realistic potential. Additional degrees are secondary qualifications and are only valuable if directly contributory to attaining new knowledge and expanding your managerial perspective.

Self-directed instruction, including computer-assisted instruction (CAI), is another type of formal education. With the computer age in full swing, self-directed educational packages are very user-friendly and available from many fine education organizations. Check with your human resource department or, if yours is a larger facility, your educational department for suggestions on good self-directed packages.

Finally, the fifth type of formal learning is organization-sponsored programming seminars and other programs sponsored by your organization and provided for all its healthcare managers and staff. It is a good idea to attend as many of these programs as possible; you can learn as much from the dialogue among your fellow participants as you can from the instructor. Listen carefully to all questions, and engage in conversation with your colleagues following the program to get their perceptions and ways in which they might apply the material practically.

Experience-Based Learning

The third means of management development is that of experience-based learning. Experiential learning is the result of learning **on the job**. Suggestions for experienced-based learning include being attuned to the lessons of trial and error, being open to the benefits of mentoring, and practicing what you've learned—all the while keeping notes on what has worked and what has not.

The first experienced-based application is that of **trial and error**. As discussed previously in this chapter, this is simply the experience of your practical application of knowledge and learning how successful it might be. Remember to use **the I-formula from the previous chapter** in trying new ideas, reinvestigate what went wrong and what went right about your previous experience, and fine-tune your efforts accordingly.

Mentoring is yet another experience-based application, which is defined as one individual acting as a primary source of instruction for another individual. Mentoring can take place on a short-term basis, perhaps with a specific project or particular area of expertise or it can be a continuous process, such as the first year of a manager's initiation into a supervisory position. Adherence to the mentoring guidelines presented later in this chapter can be most helpful.

Other experience-based educational process includes practical application of the knowledge you've gained in a realistic setting. Once again, use of your ever-present notebook is important, so that you can record many new processes you have now tried and mastered and notate what was learned from each experience.

Experience-based learning also includes your participation in the activities of a team, of which you are a part but not necessarily the leader. Collate information on what the team has achieved, what it has learned, and what you would do if you were the team leader. This will allow you to focus on the objectives and processes you will need as a team leader.

Two additional sources of experience-based learning are primary exposure and secondary-effect education. Primary exposure is the culmination of basic experiences you participated in and were a major agent for taking action. Secondary-effect education is the process by which you have learned from the triumphs and mistakes of others and have notated these accordingly.

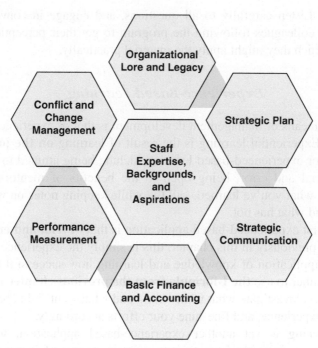

FIGURE 9–2.   Seven focus areas for new healthcare leader learning.

Numerous areas of expertise should be available to you within your organization for your own management development. Figure 9–2 identifies areas that are particularly important as you make the transition into healthcare management. Methods of acquiring these specific attributes and competencies are suggested through this book's practical resources. Use Figure 9–2 not only as a review of the material in this section, but also as your own individual development plan as you experience what might be the most educational year of your life—your first year as a healthcare manager. The individual development plan will be discussed in further detail in the following section.

STAFF AND EMPLOYEE DEVELOPMENT

Of equal importance to your own development as a manager is the development of the staff and employees who report directly to you. As stated earlier in this chapter, training is essential to staff morale, individual motivation, and maximization of employee potential. As a manager, you are responsible for the training and development of all your assigned subordinates. Because of a dearth of training and development activities due to budget cuts and other factors, it is incumbent on you to provide staff training and development.

Many benefits can be derived from your acting as the major proponent of training and development for your staff. By instructing or facilitating a seminar or teaching an in-service program, you can increase your own presentation skills and public speaking skills. Although many people fear public speaking, it is essential to your own management development to achieve a certain comfort level in this area. By acting as a trainer for your assigned staff, you can achieve this objective.

Training provides other benefits to the manager. The more your staff is trained, the greater their level of competence and the higher their achievement level in all performance activities. A major objective of any department is to develop **bench strength**, a term that relates to the ability to have depth of talent across your entire department. Each strength is achieved by having a diversity of talent and individual strengths. Obviously, this can be enhanced by training and development throughout your group.

One of the most important things a manager must do initially in his or her new role is to establish credibility. Given that you have a certain degree of technical aptitude, as well as basic communication skills, you have a tremendous base from which to develop initial credibility. By training your staff members on a group, individual, or cross-training basis, you are demonstrating your knowledge as well as your dedication to their development. When you conduct group training, you help enhance team building. When you work with individuals on a one-on-one basis, you set a strong norm that shows your willingness to accept their ideas, your interest in their development, and your readiness to establish a work relationship based on communication and trust. When you cross-train your staff, you emphasize work role flexibility.

Implementing an Individual Development Plan

The individual development plan (IDP) is a sound tool for establishing a group training program (see sample in Figure 9–3). The plan identifies specific training needs for each staff member, as well as activities that address each need.

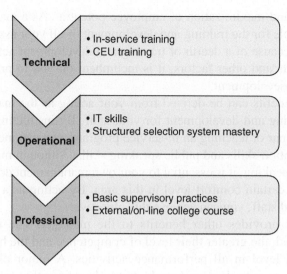

FIGURE 9–3. Individual Development Plan (IDP) sample: annual IDP for a nurse recruiter.

Start this process by, first noting the individual's name, his or her current position and starting date, the date on which the IDP is being completed, and your own name as supervisor/manager. Next, write down specific training needs identified for each individual in the department, followed by the activity that should be undertaken to fulfill the training need, the estimated time the training should take place, the learning value of each training activity, and any comments related to the activity. This is a relatively straightforward tool and should be completed every year with a maximum of five objectives filled in for each individual.

Several procedures should be followed to ensure efficacy of the IDP. A logical starting point for establishing a training and development strategy is to perform a needs analysis. A **needs analysis** explores the strengths and weaknesses of all individuals within your department and projects a training plan on both an individual and a group basis. The exploration involves a comparison of individual strengths and weaknesses with basic areas in which you expect each team member to have a certain degree of proficiency. For example, areas of competency would include the basic nursing skills required of a floor nurse, the ability on the part of the pharmacist to fill prescriptions accurately, the ability of a recruiter to interview and select individuals, and so on.

Once the basic areas of competency have been identified, you will then conduct a basic inventory of the present skills of your team members and ascertain what direction their training should fellow. To do this inventory, first review the prior performance records of each employee, including any training records that might be on file, as well as the performance evaluation and appraisals from prior years. If possible, discuss with your predecessor each individual's strengths and weaknesses, and take notes. Then assess your observation of each individual's strengths and weaknesses in comparison to the information provided.

The second step is to sit with each individual and have a candid conversation of his or her strengths and weaknesses. The best way to conduct this conversation is not to use the words' strengths and weaknesses but basically ask each employee "What type of training are you interested in?" Probe further by asking what areas he or she would like to improve in, what technical abilities to enhance, and what new areas are of interest. The net effect of this conversation should have enough data to complete the IDP effectively.

When using the IDP form, try to establish training goals and activities jointly. Ask for suggestions for what type of training might be undertaken, and what types of programs might be good for candidates. Always remember to use your human resource and educational departments whenever possible; they are experts in identifying training areas and usually have good data on what programs are effective and easily applicable.

A very important entry on the IDP form is that of estimated time of completion. Assigning a training goal is one thing—accomplishing the training needed is another. Make sure that you put a time range of 1 to 2 months (eg, March-April 2014) so that the individual can realistically address the training need on a timely basis.

Also discuss with each staff member the outcome of all training endeavors. Following their attendance at a training program, sit with each staff member and ask the following questions:

What were three major things that you learned?

Would you recommend the program to others?

On a scale of 1 to 5, how would you rate the learning value of the program (1 being highest value)?

What things did you learn that each of us here in the department can learn from?

By asking these questions, and perhaps using an evaluation form covering the program quality, you can build a data bank not only on the individual's proficiency but on the strength of the training program. This will help you in assigning training goals for other individuals and give you a natural follow-up strategy with the individual's development program.

Planning for Similar Group Needs

As you undertake the training and development process, specifically the needs analysis and other IDP functions, you will find that many individuals have similar needs throughout your department. Therefore, use a group IDP form as depicted in Figure 9–4. Simply enter the names of individuals who have common training needs, the event, the time, and the follow-up strategy you will undertake to ensure learning value. This might include a group discussion with the individuals who took the program or a series of one-on-one conversations to determine independently the quality of the program. Coordinating training needs in an economical use of time and money gives you a synergistic effect, as the individuals attending the same or similar programs will learn from each other as well as from the program leaders.

In establishing IDPs, make sure that you look to programs that are practical and will address specific needs. Do not try to overload individuals with training—3 to 5 training activities per year is about right given

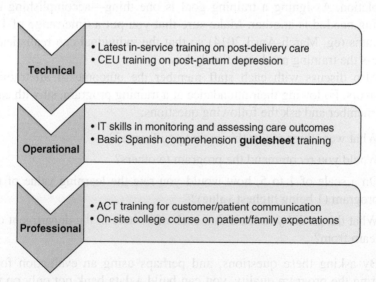

FIGURE 9–4.   Group Development Plan (GDP) sample: new baby unit of a community hospital.

today's healthcare climate and workplace conditions. Remember that training activities do not necessarily have to be restricted to workshops. Many individuals in your department, specifically those on your staff, can learn from the same sources of learning presented earlier in this chapter. Remember, however, that just as each individual has a different personality, he or she also has a different aptitude for learning and is interested in different agendas. Therefore, do not expect individuals to learn the same material in the same way, with the result. There might be common perceptions about the quality of the program, but the net yield will always be different. Take the time to understand each individual's particular training needs, as well as the effect and outcome of each learning experience.

SERVING AS AN EDUCATOR

Many times in your career as a healthcare manager you will be asked to act as a trainer for a certain program. Furthermore, there will be many opportunities to present training and educational materials to your own staff. Therefore, it is important to have a basic understanding of the dynamics of training and to take a look at some parameters for success.

Preparing for the Training Session

Good training is only as good as the preparation that goes into the program. A smart trainer analyzes the group from several perspectives. First, take a look at individual personalities; determine who your **talkers** are and who your **listeners** are. Then try to determine how motivated the group is toward the training. Individuals will be motivated to training depending on the topic. Get a realistic grip on what the level of motivation might be, and plan your strategy accordingly. If the topic is **dry**, you might want to prepare a couple of videos. If it is a topic that lends itself to discussion, you might want to **prepare some pertinent questions** so that you can lead a guided discussion about the topic.

Prepare your material in a general-to-specific context. Simply outline your text material in a general sense, and underscore points that are of specific relevance. Try to make your presentation as logical as possible, and allow yourself enough time to cover each point as fully as possible. A good rule of thumb is to provide a new idea every five minutes if you are doing a one-hour presentation. Given this scheme, four major topics, with three subtopics (or primary points) each, would constitute a solid hour of training. Try to stay within these parameters as you establish a training plan.

Always prepare a training plan with time and events for your own reference as well as for the participants. Clearly outline your objectives in the training plan, and set a time sequence with general points of reference. This will clarify your training outcomes, the content, as well as your objectives for the program. This also gets the group involved and lets them know that the training session is for a common cause, not a didactic exercise.

Make certain that your materials are fully prepared. Any handouts should be free to typographical errors, written clearly, and free of jargon the participants are not likely to understand. Handouts should include slides and other print information you will refer to; statistics; articles, and journal pieces that support the points in topic; and anything else that might be valuable to the participants. It is better to err on the side of more than on the side of less; that means making the handout material as full and as rich as possible so that the participants can get maximum yield from the material. Time is precious to all healthcare professionals, so the training program will be seen as a waste of time unless pertinent information is provided. Make certain that the handout material is clearly formatted, well organized, and related to the topic at hand.

When you have completed your preparation, conduct a final check of all the material. **Ask yourself the following questions:**

Is the presentation logical?

Would I be able to follow the flow of information?

What questions would I ask if I were a participant?

How would I answer the questions?

What essential points should the participant walk away with?

How can I make this an interesting presentation?

Did I leave anything out?

Did I allow myself enough time?

What questions can I use to get started?

Which individuals should I target for conversation and questions?

By answering these questions, you will ensure that your preparation is completed. Remember that there are no perfect answers to any of these questions. If you have an answer that you feel comfortable with for each question, you are probably well prepared for the training.

Conducting the Training Session

There are several points to remember as you conduct the training session. First, allow members of the group to introduce themselves, giving their name, their department, how long they have been at the institution, and why they are interested in the program. If individuals are not interested in the program, ask them what they know about the session and what they might want to contribute.

Always make sure that you check out the physical parameters of the room. Whenever possible, try to use a **U-shaped configuration**. This allows individuals the opportunity to talk to each other, and it facilitates a good roundtable discussion.

Announce the time parameters of the program and make sure that the first page of the handout material shows you time and events sequence. State your learning objectives right at the beginning of the program, but following introductions.

Make mental notes of what each individual has stated as his or her interest in the program. Focus on those who express interest, using their comments beginning momentum for the program. Discount any negativity right at the beginning of the session; there will be certain individuals who do not actively engage in the program no matter what you do. **Play to the stronger participants, those who are truly interested.** This will help you get the attention of those with average or marginal interest. If you can capture the very interested and the passively interested, you have probably captured a good 80% of the group. This is a great victory, no matter what level of training you might conduct or how long you have been doing group sessions.

Utilize as many learning devices as possible in the training program. These include **case studies, videos, group discussion, and, by all means, practical applications**. Get individuals to focus on the effect that the program's topic might have on their individual work lives. Utilize the expertise of individuals in the education department or colleagues and peers who have conducted training programs previously. They might have good materials on the topic, as well as some insights on the participants and how you might deliver the program. Pace the program smartly so that you cover all material. Handle questions advantageously, for example, repeat the question back to the inquirer, state what your position might be, and always ask the entire group the question and what their thoughts might be. Usually the answer—in fact, the best answer lies somewhere among the participants.

Closing the Training Session

Close with a practical exercise. This might be a final case study or anything that recaps the material in your session.

Try to incorporate evaluations into the closing portion of the program. Allow time to critique the program relative to subject, delivery, applicability, and whether participants would refer the program as a sound training exercise to other individuals. **Do not take criticism personally.** Try to be objective, and use the participation in the program, the usage of your material, and the attitude of the participants as your true measures of success. Constantly upgrade the program by adding to it and garnering suggestions from participants.

Finally, recognize that the more you conduct training, the better you will become at it. You will also find that you, more than any of your participants, learn from the programs. By combining these two factors, as well as incorporating the information in this section, conducting training programs will become an important and enjoyable part of your management arsenal.

Mentoring and Delegation

Two overlooked but practical strategies for developing and educating staff are mentoring and delegation. **Mentoring** refers to the one-on-one educational process of an experienced individual teaching an inexperienced (or less experienced) individual a certain procedure or set of skills. **Delegation** is the assignment of a specific task in the interest of expedience of action and learning. This section will cover both, including their pitfalls and strengths as management techniques.

Role of the Mentor

Mentoring should be based on the establishment of objectives for the individual being mentored. The mentor should sit down with the individual and establish specific areas of need. The mentor should also identify areas of potential and perceived needs that the employee might not be aware of. For example, the human resource professional might need expertise in hiring and selection; the mentor might suggest that the budgeting process inherent to these responsibilities is equally important.

As always, liaison should be established with the education department, the human resource department, and perhaps the reporting manager. All of these parties should contribute their expertise as well as suggestions on how the mentoring process could be more efficient. Fundamentally, **mentoring takes four forms:**

1. **Activity observations:** By observing the mentor completing a particular task, an individual learns how to complete the task and has the opportunity to ask questions and to fine-tune his or her approach.

2. **A Joint Education Activity:** Both the mentor and employee can undertake an educational program in which the mentor has more experience. Subsequent to the educational activity, the mentor can specifically point out areas the employee can benefit from and respond to any questions specific to the educational exercise.

3. **Delegation:** As will be seen in the second half of this section, the mentor can indeed be the individual who delegates a specific task to the employee.

4. **Understudying:** The mentor simply guides the employees through a variety of activities as the employee observes the activities, takes part at the discretion of the mentor, and enjoys close communication and education.

The most important thing about any mentoring process is the follow-up strategy. If mentoring relationship is established over a long period of time, for example, 6 months to 1 year, it is good to have a **first Friday session**. This might entail a visit to a local restaurant or a meeting in the mentor's office to discuss the month's activities. If it is a short-term relationship, the mentor should use some of the questions contained in The Practical Resource Section to ensure that learning is taking place.

Delegation of Responsibility

Although mentoring is extremely popular today, delegation might be an even more effective strategy. As a manager, it is imperative that you delegate as many responsibilities as possible while maintaining responsibility for the ultimate outcome of the project. Figure 9–5 reviews four basic delegation guidelines. Review all four critical areas and follow the checklist in Figure 9–5 to ensure that the delegation process is fruitful.

In assigning the task, whenever possible identify assignments that are not routine. In other words, do not limit your list of **delegatable** assignments to the things that bore you, things you do not like, or things you would like to do but you have never undertaken. It is impossible to delegate what you yourself have never done and thus have no frame of reference as to how to pursue the objective.

Review the learning value inherent in each delegated task and be certain to stress this to the employee when you assign the task. Meetings, paperwork,

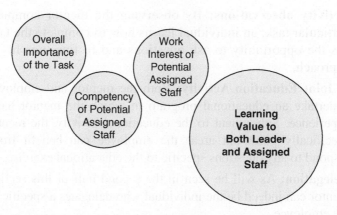

FIGURE 9–5.   Delegation guidelines.

audit activities, investigative work, and people-intensive activities are all things that can and should be delegated to increase the skills of your employees and staff.

As identified in Figure 9–6, there are two types of individuals to whom you will find yourself delegating tasks. The first is the **go-to** individual, the person who has done the task a variety of times and has achieved total competency but derives little learning value because he or she has achieved mastery of the task. The other individual is the **MSF (maximum stretch factor)** person. This individual has no competency in the activity or task and thus can learn up to 100% of the learning value of the task. If you have the time, you always use the MSF person, as he or she will learn and grow from the experience. This will also free up the go-to person to undertake a

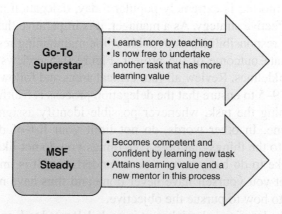

FIGURE 9–6.   The **Go-To** superstar and the MSF steady.

new assignment replete with high learning value, which would teach a new competency, as delineated in Figure 9–6.

In assigning the delegated objective, you have three choices. You could tell the individual how to do the task, which will certainly guarantee a clear outcome but limit creativity and ownership of the task. You could ask the individual how he or she wants to do the task, but without a frame of reference he or she might be unable to answer this question.

The third option is perhaps the best. Suggest to the individual how you have completed this task before; how others might have completed the task before; what a journal article had to say about handling such an assignment; and, finally, but most important, how the individual might perceive pursuing the objective. In any event, always clarify the method the individual will be using by asking specifically "How will you go about this?"

Finally, **always utilize an appropriate follow-up strategy**. Establish significant interim benchmarks to follow employee progress, and assign the objective using time, money, percentages, and numbers. Use an appropriate follow-up strategy that is keyed to the individual's personality. If he or she is somewhat dependent on you, you might want to simply tell them to follow up with you whenever they feel the need. In any event, remember to keep abreast of any developments and progress toward the goal by checking in with employee on a regular basis.

After assigning the goal and delegating the task, keep notes either in your calendar, in a set of files for each employee, or in a notebook to ensure that you are informed of the employee's progress. Always ask the individual what he or she is learning from the task, and underscore this by discussing the learning value upon conclusion of the task.

As a new healthcare manager, you will find yourself being the delegatee and mentoree more often than the delegator or mentor. It is important, however, to try these skills to incorporate them into your everyday activities. Not only are they sound management devices, their development value cannot be overstated.

SUMMARY

The role of a teacher is intrinsic to the healthcare leader's everyday responsibilities. Every day is not only an opportunity to learn, but an opportunity to teach and educate. The successful fulfillment of both roles contributes mightily to the ultimate success of a healthcare organization.

PRACTICAL RESOURCE—CHAPTER IX:
Strategic Guidesheets

This set of guidesheets is intended to reinforce your management action and leadership acumen in critical situations. This resource is intended to assist you in **asking the right questions** to both yourself and appropriate staff members and other organizational players involved in these situations. The guidesheets have been grouped categorically so that you can access them quickly.

Group I: Making the Transition: First Management Steps
Management orientation guide

Assessing your team's prior performance

Leadership model identification

Diagnosing individual motivational tendencies

Group II: Hiring, Counseling, and Firing
Conducting a job description review

Establishing a candidate's **Wish List**

Making a timely hiring decision

Counseling guide for the chronic poor performer

Reviewing individual performance with a staff member

Validating performance documentation

Conducting the performance evaluation session

Termination considerations

Group III: Personal/Self-Management Techniques
Meeting participation preparation

Meeting management preparation

Stress management checklist

Maximizing the relationship with your supervisor

Time management consideration

Group IV: Critical Management Applications
Crisis management guidelines

Resolving workplace conflict

Planning and managing change effectively

Reviewing decision-making criteria

Action planning guidelines

Preparing a critical communication message

Clear assignment of delegated tasks: questions to ask the delegate

Clear reception of delegated assignments

Group V: Staff Education and Development

Conducting a staff educational needs analysis

Seminar presentation checklist

Staff education preparation

Seminar participation preparation

Utilize the material in this appendix as mandated by the situation. Remember also to use the other pertinent questions throughout the text that might also help you manage critical situations.

Group I: Making the Transition: First Management Steps
Management Orientation Guide

1. Do I understand the entire organization mission and set of values for healthcare delivery?

2. Have I discussed fully my supervisor's expectations for my department and assigned resources?

3. Do I understand what my supervisor expects from me as a member of his/her management team?

4. What have I learned about my predecessor in this position that is positive and can be built on?

5. What have I learned about my predecessor's activities or management style that was negative and should be avoided?

6. Who among my staff do I expect to be great performers and role models within the department?

7. Who among the staff are my steady players and appear to be the core of the work group?

8. Who among the work group are poor performers and likely to create performance problems?

9. What objectives are important personally to me in my first year of healthcare management?

10. What objectives do I want my staff to achieve in my first year as their manager?

Assessing Your Team's Prior Performance

1. What adjectives did your supervisor use to describe your depart-ment during your orientation and selection process?

2. What input did colleagues give your relative to your group's performance and past history?

3. Who in the group was cited as being a **strong player?**

4. Who was cited as being a **problem player?**

5. What was reflected in the individual performance evaluations of the group members?

6. What knowledge, if any, has personally collected at the outset of your leadership of the group?

7. What reasons were given for your predecessor's departure?

8. In your initial opinion, did your predecessor do a good, average, or poor job managing the group?

9. What mistakes did your predecessor make in managing the group that you will seek to avoid?

10. Given all of the above, what four general statements would you make about your group's performance?

    a.

    b.

    c.

    d.

11. What three actions will you take to activate positive group perfor-mance, including things your predecessor did that you will or will not do?

    a.

    b.

    c.

Leadership Model Identification

1. Considering my upbringing, who were the major positive influences on my life in general?

2. Considering my upbringing, who were the major models for my leadership and interpersonal communication style?

3. Who are some historical leaders I admire?

4. What are some traits that I admire in the historical and popular leaders that I might try out in my efforts?

5. Who are the best **bosses** I've had?

6. What qualities among my previous supervisors did I admire and might I try out?

7. What are some incidents or events that I saw were handled particularly well by a leader? What was the lesson for me?

8. What were some major failings of some poor leaders from history? How can I avoid the same mistakes?

9. Considering organizational and professional leaders I've observed, what are some major mistakes they made that I will avoid?

10. If I had to use five adjectives to describe the leadership style I aspire to, the description would be:

    a.

    b.

    c.

    d.

    e.

Analyzing Work Group Morale

1. What four adjectives would I use to describe the collective attitude of my department when I took command?

    a.

    b.

    c.

    d.

2. Why do I think the prevailing attitude of the work group corresponded to those four adjectives?

3. What major factors in the work environment trigger an attitudinal reaction in my work group?

4. Which of these factors from question 3 are within my control as a manager to change positively?

5. Which of these factors is somewhat out of my control as the group's manager?

6. Which members of my staff are usually positive and have a strong positive effect on the attitudes of the rest of the group?

7. Which members of my group have chronically negative attitude and have a dragging effect on other members of the group?

8. How can I reinforce the positive actions and attitudes of the individual(s) cited in question 6?

9. How can I constructively diminish the negative effects of the attitudes of the individual(s) cited in question 7?

10. What additional measures can I take in creating a higher level of positive morale within my work group?

Diagnosing Individual Motivational Tendencies

1. The three most positively motivated members of my staff are:

   a.

   b.

   c.

2. These three individuals can be described (using adjectives) as:

   a.

   b.

   c.

3. The three most negatively motivated individuals in my department are:

   a.

   b.

   c.

4. I would describe these individuals as:

   a.

   b.

   c.

5. The performance level of the positively motivated individuals is:*

   a. Above average to outstanding

   b. Satisfactory/average

   c. Below average

6. The performance level of the negatively motivated individuals is:*

   a. Above average

   b. Satisfactory

   c. Below average

---

*Rate performance relative to all 3 collectively or individually.

7. The major positive motivating force for the positive performers is:

_____ .

8. The major negative factor the poor performers **harp about** is:

_____ .

9. I will encourage the positively motivated individuals by:
   a.
   b.
   c.
10. I will address the negatively motivated individuals by:
    a. Counseling
    b. Performance evaluation
    c. Beginning the documentation to termination process

Group II: Hiring, Counseling, and Firing
Conducting a Job Description Review

1. Does the current job description reflect at least 75% of the major responsibilities of the position in a general sense?

2. Does the current job description show accurately about 75% of the time quotient of a typical day for a person in the position?

3. Does the current job description show major factors that would be considered vitally successful in the normal conduct of the job position?

4. Does the job description present all current applicable ADA—and/or EEOC—mandated information?

5. Does the current job description list more than 12 responsibilities that are deemed **major**? Can some of these be combined?

6. Does the current job description appear outdated because it does not include several major current responsibilities?

7. What significant incidents (ie, action beyond or below the norm) and critical contributions should be on the job description or at least considered in the hiring process?

8. Are the primary educational and experiential requisites of the job position clearly enumerated on the job description?

9. What improvements should be made to the job description to make it a viable management tool?

10. What factors not present on the job description should be considered in the hiring process?

Establishing a Candidate's Wish List

1. What technical abilities should the ideal candidate for this position possess?

2. What key interpersonal characteristics should the ideal candidate possess, considering the basic interpersonal interaction required in this position?

3. What technical and interpersonal characteristics did the best performers in this position exemplify?

4. What negative technical and/or interpersonal characteristics did the worst performers in this position demonstrate?

5. What characteristics do other members of my team think would be beneficial in this position?

6. What characteristics would my staff consider definitely detrimental in this position?

7. What input has my supervisor provided in considering the ideal tenets for this particular position?

8. Considering current staff demands and goals, what specific skills or characteristics would be ideal in this position?

9. Considering future goals and dynamics affecting the organization and my department, what characteristics should the ideal candidate possess?

10. My gut instinct and professional expertise tell me that the best available candidate for this position would possess the following three characteristics and three technical abilities:

Characteristics:	Abilities:
a.	a.
b.	b.
c.	c.

Making a Timely Hiring Decision

1. Of the available pool of candidates, is this candidate the best qualified in terms of technical expertise?

2. Did the candidate display a consistently sound attitude in all of my interaction with him/her throughout the interview process?

3. Does the candidate have strong listening and perceiving skills, as evidenced by his/her interview interaction?

4. Did the candidate seem truly comfortable in his/her interactions throughout the interview process?

5. Was the candidate comfortable and confident in describing past experiences and work achievement?

6. Were the perceptions of other individuals in the selection process—my supervisor, colleagues, and staff members—generally favorable and enthusiastic?

7. Do I have any strong reservations about the candidate (a major performance liability we'll have to work on)?

8. Will this person fit into the current work group as a positive force and source of motivation and technical expertise?

9. Does this person fully understand the job and have realistic expectations of what the job will entail on a daily basis?

10. Did the person ask reasonable questions appropriately throughout the interviewing process?

11. Is my level of comfort with the individual reasonably high relative to his/her potential and probable performance in this job?

Counseling Guide for the Chronic Poor Performer

1. Is all of my documentation accurate and objective?

2. Does my documentation contain clear facts—dates, times, and events—that illustrate the poor performance?

3. What is the significant effect of this type of performance on the overall staff and work group?

4. What is the specific effect of this type of performance on the delivery of health care to the customer/patient?

5. How does this poor performance affect the entire organization's ability to provide top-notch health care?

6. How quickly do I want this performance to be remedied and completely turned around?

7. How will both the performer and I know when this performance is corrected to my expectation?

8. Will this person fit into the current work group as a positive force and source of motivation and technical expertise?

9. Does this person fully understand the job and have realistic expectations of what the job will entail on a daily basis?

10. Did the person ask reasonable questions appropriately throughout the interviewing process?

11. Is my level of comfort with the individual reasonably high relative to his/her potential and probable performance in this job?

Reviewing Individual Performance with a Staff Member

1. Have I reviewed all of my documentation notes thoroughly and objectively as possible?

2. What conversations have I had with this staff member that might be used as a constructive reference in this conversation?

3. Have I kept this person's current performance by consistent feedback and timely performance direction?

4. How has this person's performance objectives changed over the past year?

5. What significant contributions has this person made over the past grading period that are truly noteworthy?

6. What critical incidents has this person handled successfully over the course of the past year?

7. Has the person failed to deliver expected performance relative to a critical incident?

8. What kind of evaluation does this person probably expect, and is he/she justified in that expectation?

9. What major performance objectives have I quantified for the next year for this individual?

10. What training and development activities does this person want to pursue that I consider progressive?

11. What potential significant incidents (ie, new job responsibilities and so forth) do I foresee on the horizon for this person's job position?

Validating Performance Documentation

1. Am I keeping current documentation on all the members of my staff?
2. Are the entries in my logbook, both positive and negative in nature, reflective of the work performance documented?
3. Do I have an appropriate number of entries on all the members of my staff?
4. Are numbers, financial designations, time quotients, and percentages used as much as possible to depict performance entries?
5. Is each performance entry immediately followed by counseling session, which is then recorded?
6. Has chronic poor performance been recorded, counseled, and presented directly to the poor performer for correction?
7. Has strong positive performance been recorded and presented to the individual in the interest of expressing appreciation, encouraging motivation, and encouraging progressive development?
8. Am I basically comfortable with the entries in terms of:
   a. Fairness?
   b. Accuracy?
   c. Detail?
   d. Objectivity?
9. Is the entire range of documentation being fully used to increase the quality of overall staff performance?
10. Is the documentation being used individually in the construction of individual performance evaluation?

Conducting the Performance Evaluation Session

1. Have I asked the performer ahead of time to suggest critical contributions and significant incident management examples that I might have missed?

2. Have I asked the performer a month before the session to compile a list of desired training and development activities?

3. Are all of the ratings fair and substantiated?

To the Reviewed Staff Member:

4. Do you understand my explanations of the ratings and the rationale and data supporting the ratings?

5. What questions do you have about the evaluation in general or relative to specific elements or sections?

6. What resources do you need to get even better in your work position?

7. What can I do to better assist your work efforts in the coming grading period?

8. What types of work activity would you like to become involved in the next year that might be new and different for you?

9. What 3 training and development activities do you want to pursue in the next year?

   a.

   b.

   c.

10. What type of training, development, or direct education do you need to receive the next year to maximize your performance?

Termination Considerations

1. What is the effect of the poor performer(s) on the rest of my staff?
2. What are some of the problems the poor performer(s) causes considering overall staff achievement?
3. What documentation exists currently on this poor performer in the employee file (including performance evaluations and other significant data)?
4. What documentation have I established about this individual on his/her poor performance?
5. What efforts have I made to counsel this person and affect a turn-around in performance?
6. Has the person made a full-fledged effort to improve performance per my suggestion?
7. Is the person's poor performance evident to customers/patients, as evidenced by complaints or documentation of poor performance?
8. Have I discussed this with other managers and colleagues whose opinions I trust and value? What were their perceptions?
9. Have I discussed this with my supervisor? What guidance and input did I receive relative to this situation?
10. Trusting the answers to all of these questions, as well as my gut instincts, what odds would I give this individual to completely evolve into a strong, positive employee?

    a. 2 to 1 in favor of performance
    b. 50 to 50 (even money)
    c. 2 to 1 against turnaround
    d. 5 to 1 against turnaround

(*Key*: In question 10, anything less than the first option **2 to 1 in favor**— means that termination should be considered.)

Group III: Personal/Self-Management Techniques
Meeting Participation Preparation

1. Why was I invited to this meeting?
2. Should my participation be active/talking or passive/listening?
3. How does the meeting discussion affect me and my staff?
4. What questions do I want to ask and what pertinent information do I want to glean from the meeting?
5. What expectations do I feel the meeting's leader hold relative to my participation?
6. What prework should I complete prior to the meeting?
7. What materials or data should I bring to the meeting?
8. Who are the most prominently important players who will attend this meeting, and how can I support their agenda?
9. How can I make the strongest contribution possible within the context of this meeting?
10. What potentially valuable information can I gain from this meeting that might benefit me and my staff?

Meeting Management Preparation

1. What is the specific intent of the meeting, and what is the desired outcome?
2. Have I invited all the appropriate members of my staff to this meeting and tactfully eliminated any nonessential participation?
3. Has appropriate prework been assigned to all participants in the interest of maximizing the meeting's conduct?
4. Does everyone involved know what time the meeting starts and how long it will last?
5. What type of leadership style do I want to impart throughout the conduct of the meeting?
6. What specific questions do I want to ask the attendees in order to get optimum participation?
7. How much participation do I want from the group in general relative to the topic and desired outcome?
8. Who are the major players relative to the meeting's topic and have ensured their active participation?
9. What major themes do I want to present in the meeting, and what 3 key points do I want to highlight?
10. What 3 next steps do I want to see acted on as practical, tangible outcomes of the meeting?

Stress Management Checklist

1. What on-the-job methods will I maintain to decrease the negative effects of stress?

2. What off-the-job methods will I incorporate into my lifestyle to negate the negative effects of stress?

3. My first 5+ day vacation is scheduled for _____.

4. My second 5+ day vacation for this year (might include weekend) is scheduled for _____.

5. To combat negative stress, I will pursue my favorite physical fitness activity of _____ at least twice a week.

6. To combat negative stress, I will pursue my favorite avocation/hobby of _____ at least once a week.

7. For every 2 hours of intense work, I take a 5-to-10-minute break.

8. Which members of my staff tend to work hard rather than smart?

9. Have I counseled the individuals cited in question 8 and encouraged them to take stress-positive measures?

10. Have I properly explained the demands of healthcare management and enlisted the aid of my family and friends in maintaining a healthy balance?

Maximizing the Relationship with Your Supervisor

1. What primary goals for my first 3 months does my supervisor expect from me?

2. What first-year objectives does my supervisor hold for my efforts as a manager and management team member?

3. What style does my supervisor utilize, and what aspects of that style have potential merit in my efforts?

4. Have my supervisor and I established a plan to meet at least once a month to discuss key objectives and goals?

5. Have my supervisor and I established a standard operating procedure for resolving crisis and critical management events?

6. What specific aspects of my supervisor's professional background have potential professional development value for me?

7. Have I taken every opportunity to review key events with my supervisor to get appropriate advice and learning insight?

8. Have I taken every opportunity to educate my supervisor to the particular dynamics of my new management responsibilities?

9. What long-range goals does my supervisor have and how do I contribute to making those aspirations become reality?

10. What organizational goals and mission objectives are most important for my supervisor and me to periodically discuss?

Time Management Considerations

1. What are the major problems I have in managing my time?

2. What problems do I create for myself by not properly managing my time efficiently?

3. Which parts of my responsibilities could I possibly manage more efficiently (eg, communication, mail, and meetings)?

4. Would the stoplight method work in handling at least one of my responsibilities? If so, which one(s)?

5. Would setting a priority or importance rating to some of my responsibilities be helpful? If so, which one(s)?

6. Would a filing system or assigned desk drawer system assist in managing some responsibilities?

7. Who among my staff has difficulty managing their time? How can I assist them and which system should they use to increase their time efficiency?

8. Which supervisors throughout my career seemed to manage their time poorly? Why did this occur, and how should they have remedied the problem?

9. Who among my previous supervisors were good time managers? What were some of their **secrets of success** in this regard?

10. From the outset of my management career, what commitments to time management, either formally using a system or informally in organizing work, will I employ?

Group IV: Critical Management Applications

Crisis Management Guidelines

1. What is the paramount crisis at hand, in specific detail?

2. What major effect does the crisis have on my entire work group and staff?

3. What less apparent effects does the crisis have on my work group and staff?

4. What have the initial reactions to the crisis been by the entire staff?

5. Who among my staff seems to be the most severely affected at the outset of the crisis?

6. Up to now, who among my staff knows about the crisis and its negative effects?

7. What are the major fears among my staff regarding crisis and its negative effects?

8. What are the major fears of my staff?

9. What suggestions have I sought and received from my staff regarding a positive response to the crisis?

10. What plan of action have we innovated, endorsed, and accepted as being the best reaction to the crisis at hand?

Resolving Workplace Conflict

1. What is the major conflict as defined by the players?
2. What is the major conflict in my perception?
3. Which individuals are most involved in the conflict?
4. Who is virtually unaffected by the conflict?
5. Have I had a specific conversation with the individuals cited in question 3?
6. Have I tactfully eliminated from the conflict the players indicated in question 4?
7. Is the conflict created by interpersonal relationship?
8. Is the conflict created by work dynamics I can control?
9. Have I stated my expectations for professionalism to both parties?
10. Have I conducted a conversation focused on suggestions from the conflicted participants on how to resolve the conflict?
11. Have I requested help from other appropriate professionals (eg, my supervisor or the human resource department)?
12. Have I settled on a specific solution and demanded compliance from both parties?

Planning and Managing Change Effectively

1. Will the change positively affect the status quo?
2. What are the major benefits of the change, as I perceive them as manager and group leader?
3. What major benefit, if any, does my staff perceive as being effected by the change?
4. Is my staff basically supportive of this change? Why or why not?
5. Is my staff basically resistive to this change? Why or why not? (possibilities: fear, apprehension, stress, too much change too fast, and skepticism)
6. What short-term problems has my staff identified as being potential problems in implementing the change?
7. What solutions to these problems have both my staff and I discussed in meetings or one-on-one?
8. What long-term benefits have my staff and I identified in implementing this change?
9. How will this change benefit the department?
10. How will this change benefit the organization?
11. How will this change benefit the individual in my department on a person-by-person basis?

Reviewing Decision-Making Criteria

1. What major objectives will this decision help achieve in the short term?
2. What long-term benefits will this decision help accomplish that will be obvious to all parties?
3. What are some major problems that will be created by the decision?
4. What are some existing conditions that will be negatively affected by the decision?
5. How does the decision relate to our organization's objectives, mission, and values?
6. Who will be the major contributors on my staff toward making the action of the decision happen?
7. Who will be the individuals most negatively impacted by the decision?
8. What major financial considerations bear on this decision and its outcome(s)?
9. Have I considered all logical input in this decision fully and utilized available data? Should I wait for more data or act now?
10. Considering all of the data and my **gut feel**, do I:

    __ Have all the facts?

    __ Have enough information?

    __ Know that the time to act is now?

    __ Feel as comfortable as possible in acting now?

Action Planning Guidelines

1. What is the major objective of the action I'm about to undertake in terms of organization contribution?

2. What benefits will the action provide to the organization and my department's performance and accomplishment?

3. What are the perceptions of my supervisor with regard to this planned action (including suggestions and tips provided by him or her)?

4. What significant data and input have I considered that really affected my decision to take this action?

5. How can I reinforce the major reasons for taking this action throughout the entire process of change?

6. Are the major players on my staff completely aware of the intent of the action and specifically what their role(s) will be in this undertaking?

7. How will I present the major objective and subsequent action steps to appropriate members of my staff?

8. What potential problems might occur throughout the process? How might I avoid or alleviate the negative interaction of these effects?

9. Have I completely identified all of the improvements this action might bring about?

10. What are three most important action elements I should remember throughout this entire undertaking?

    a.

    b.

    c.

Preparing a Critical Communication Message

1. What is the major point that I want to get across?
2. What is the best way to get the receiver(s) interested in this message?
3. What are the important aspects of this message in my perception?
4. What are the most important aspects of this message in the receiver's perception?
5. What questions might the group ask relative to the message?
6. How might I answer the receiver's questions?
7. Are there potential opportunities for the message to become garbled or misunderstood?
8. How might I ensure that the communication is as clear as possible and direct in its effect?
9. What immediate action do I want this message to motivate?
10. How will I emphasize the message's importance, action needed, and long-range positive support of this message?

Clear Assignment of Delegated Tasks: Questions to Ask the Delegate

1. Do you understand why I selected you for this assignment? (Express confidence and stress learning value.)

2. Do you have a handle on what the finished project should be? (Provide a visualization of your expected outcome.)

3. Have I provided you with enough suggestions regarding how I have undertaken this kind of assignment?

4. What other resources might you want to consult prior to tackling this assignment?

5. Outline the financial considerations for this assignment, including expenses to be incurred and potential cost savings.

6. How much time do you think you'll need to complete this assignment at the best possible level?

7. How often do you want to meet with me to discuss your progress and the overall conduct of this assignment?

8. What calls or other types of communication do you want me to make as you conduct this project?

9. Can you think of anything we might have missed as we planned this undertaking? Have we covered all the important areas you can think of?

10. What do you think you'll learn from this whole event? (Use this question appropriately throughout the process.)

Clear Reception of Delegated Assignments

1. Why is this project or assignment being delegated to me?

2. What is the overall expected outcome of my action in carrying out this assignment?

3. What suggestions has my supervisor (or the appropriate delegator) made relative to successful completion of this assignment?

4. What resources or sources of information has my supervisor recommended for consultation regarding this assignment?

5. What resources or contacts should I consult in the interest of effectively completing this assignment?

6. Who has completed this assignment previously, and how can I benefit from their experience?

7. How will I know when I'm making progress toward my objective?

8. Have I scheduled regular follow-up sessions with the delegator to ensure that I'm on the right track?

9. Who should be involved in this process with me in order to ensure completion, considering my staff and fellow professional colleagues?

10. What are the major learning opportunities in undertaking this assignment?

Group V: Staff Education and Development

Conducting a Staff Educational Needs Analysis

1. What apparent educational needs does my entire staff have and how does this influence performance?

2. What specific educational needs does (name of employee) have that impacts his/her performance negatively?

3. Have I discussed training, development, and educational needs with each staff member individually?

4. Have I discussed training, educational, and developmental needs with the entire group in staff meetings?

5. What types of courses are offered at the local community college, university, or adult educational unit that might benefit my staff?

6. Can all members of my staff read and write properly? If not, have they explored literacy program possibilities with the human resource department?

7. What assistance can the organization's educational department or human resource unit provide to my staff in general?

8. What specific assistance has the human resource department or education staff offered to particular staff members? Can I use them as references?

9. What types of education and training would be most effective considering available time, past success, and business demands?

10. What short-term and long-term educational needs does my staff possess that can realistically be addressed?

Seminar Presentation Checklist

1. Have I considered all of the major learning objectives fully as they relate to the overall seminar group?

2. Are my materials current in terms of technical information and vital data?

3. Have I allocated enough time for the entire presentation, including attendee participation breaks and questions?

4. Do I have appropriate visual aids and other **learning hooks** to optimize the interest quotient for the program?

5. Would I find this program interesting if I were a participant with an average interest in the topic?

6. Have I tried out the presentation with a trusted test audience (eg, spouse, colleagues, or friend)?

7. What potential questions might participants ask? What answers might provide maximum information and clarification?

8. Who among the group will be extremely supportive of the information and the seminar conduct?

9. Who among the group might detract or counter the information unfairly? Do I have strategies prepared to get them back on track?

10. Have I stressed the benefit and importance of the information to my group prior to the program? Will I emphasize this at the outset of the program?

Staff Education Preparation

1. What major learning needs does my staff have from a general perspective that can be addressed in a group process?

2. What specific needs does each member of my staff have in terms of professional and technical expertise?

3. What forum would be best for a staff educational event, on-site or off-site, considering financial realities?

4. What style of presentation would be appropriate, considering group participation lecture or a **mixed-bag** presentation?

5. How long should the session be in order to cover all the required education points and allow appropriate time for interaction and questions?

6. Should I, as the department manager, conduct the training or should someone else facilitate the program?

7. Who is the best qualified to conduct the session in terms of professional expertise and teaching experience?

8. What references has the potential seminar leader provided? Have the references been validated by my specific questions?

9. What materials would be most applicable to our group, and what information would they find most valuable?

10. List the 3 major practical outcomes desired from the training session:

    a.

    b.

    c.

Seminar Participation Preparation

1. What is my general interest in this program?
2. What specific learning objectives do I want to achieve by attending this program?
3. What information do I want to provide to program facilitator in the conduct of the program?
4. What learning objectives do I want the seminar materials to address in order to maximize my investment in this program?
5. What major aspects of my current management role might be benefited by my attendance at this program?
6. What long-range benefit might I receive from this program?
7. What immediate benefits do I expect to receive from this program?
8. Is it likely that most of the participants will have the same learning agenda as mine?
9. What questions do I want the instructor/facilitator to specifically address?
10. What information might my fellow participants provide that I could benefit from directly?

CHAPTER TEN

Applying the C-Formula: Strategies for Staff Engagement

If the eyes are the windows to the soul, then communication is the key to action. As a healthcare leader, you will find staff engagement through communication to be linchpin to all of your activities. As we discussed generally in the preceding chapters, the strength of your communication will directly reflect the effectiveness of your performance efforts.

Communication training and development for a healthcare manager must go beyond platitudes and clichés to become a style that is both comfortable and natural and one that will provide maximum impact. It is also vital to use a communication strategy that allows you to get information on a timely basis and to provide needed work direction in an efficient manner.

This chapter will explore the essential dynamics effective to healthcare management communication and the interpersonal dynamics essential to the healthcare leader's role. The use of the title the **C-Formula** and its handy alliteration of the letter C will assist you in the practical application of proven strategies that can help you maximize the communication process with your staff and other important players in your sphere of influence. Also provided will be insight on specific communication dynamics, including written communication, group communication, and interactions between yourself and your superiors. By exploring both the virtues of good communication and the pitfalls of poor communication, this chapter will provide you with valuable guidelines as you undertake your management role.

DYNAMICS OF EFFECTIVE HEALTHCARE MANAGEMENT COMMUNICATION

In your role as a healthcare or physician leader, you must master four essential dynamics of communication: climate, community, content, and challenge. **Climate** refers here to the workplace environment, which you help define, and the overall atmosphere throughout the healthcare workplace. The term **community** as used in this chapter relates to the team orientation of your department and to the overall organization in which you work, including all lines of communication within the organization. **Content** refers to the way you deliver messages—the style, message, elements, and manner in which information is provided and direction is given. Finally, **challenge** refers to how critical communication, vital work parameters, and directives are delivered to appropriate members of the organization.

In each of these four areas, a set of essential components comprises the dynamics of communication in the healthcare environment. These components are summarized throughout the following subsections and offered as guideposts for your own approach to effective communication in your new role.

The Climate of the Work Environment

For a work climate to be prosperous and produce good results on a regular basis, a certain amount of **coaching** must take place as the leader acts as a mentor to his or her staff as a unit and as individual staff members assist one another in attaining growth and development. In effect, coaching entails encouraging others to perform better, pointing out their mistakes constructively, and providing ongoing direction as needed to all members of the department. Too much coaching (**micromanaging**) leads to a leader becoming needlessly too detail oriented by failing to allow individuals enough professional liberty. A total lack of coaching within the department will arrest staff development and, consequently, work progress.

Accordingly, a **consultative** environment must surround the work group. This involves the sharing of expertise among the staff and the provision of technical acumen by the department leader. The healthcare manager must be a leader in becoming a consultant within the department, as well as a consultant throughout the organization on key technical issues.

Technical information provided to others in the organization must be clear and direct and conveyed in a manner that will be readily understood and useful to the receiver. The risks with consultative communication are overuse of jargon or technical terms or loss of the essential message due to failure to understand the requester's needs. When acting in a consultative role, first ask a series of questions to determine the specific nature of the problem; next, determine what technical assistance the individual needs; and then provide that assistance in a clear-cut manner while pledging any further assistance as needed.

The fourth attribute of workplace climate in terms of communication is **candor**. The worst liability you can be faced with is to be perceived as a phony or as disingenuous. Strive to be forthcoming and direct in all your communication efforts. Be forthright in dealing with individuals and in providing information; let people know that you do not have all the answers in all situations and state your dedication to finding the answers to questions and the solutions to problems. By providing false or misleading information, inconsistent or inaccurate communication, or by doing anything that can be perceived as dishonest or an attempt to **con** department members, you risk being judged untrustworthy or incompetent leading to a lack of trust that could be irreversible.

The fifth element of communication in the workplace is **collaboration**. It is essential that as a team all members collaborate on common goals and objectives. Individuals must feel comfortable working together striving toward a mutually beneficial end. Stressing the individual talents of department members is a great first step for creating a spirit of collaboration. Publicly recognizing the contributions of all team members, particularly on joint efforts, is the second step toward fostering a collaborative atmosphere. The third step is to remember the axiom, **give the good news in public, but give the bad news in private**. Thus, positive gains the department has made should be shared in public, while any performance deficiencies or problems should be discussed individually in private with those involved. This approach ensures that a positive spirit is generated throughout the group and that collaboration and joint efforts are always encouraged and rewarded.

All department members should feel they are **comrades in arms**, working together, and living by the adage, "Nobody wins unless we all win." Thus, **camaraderie** is a key element of the workplace climate. Certain key words can help establish camaraderie across the department. For example, in stressing the value of working together, the word **team** and the pronoun **we** are verbal strengtheners that reinforce the virtue of camaraderie.

Without camaraderie and collaboration, groups become disjointed and the individual is focused on at the expense of the group.

As emphasized throughout this book, the focus of communication in a progressive work climate should be on identifying and implementing solutions, not constantly reiterating and exacerbating problems. The key notion in this respect is finding a **cure**, an appropriate metaphor, given that the essential mission of a healthcare organization is to seek cures. Cures must be sought for everyday problems that arise in your department. Always ask your staff's advice on how a problem might be solved. Encourage them to provide cures to problems and reward them, either verbally or tangibly, for any successful solution. Special recognition such as **employee of the month** or paid time are two examples of appropriate awards. It is imperative that the workplace climate be geared toward providing cures and that the positive generation of progressive ideas be recognized and rewarded.

Character is another essential dimension of the workplace climate and is essentially to the work personality demonstrated and embraced by all members of the department. Any communication should be delivered in a way that is thoughtful, tactful, and ethically sound. This precludes publicly berating any employee who is not performing up to standards. Thoughtful delivery also mandates the use of tactful language and appropriate courtesy when discussing key issues. Furthermore, character defines to what extent each individual in the department interrelates with dignity, class, and basic compassion. Lack of any of these positive attributes within the work climate will result in an environment that breeds discomfort, threatens individual dignity, and abets negative aspects of performance and poor team interaction that will soon surface.

Change takes place in the healthcare environment every day. The clear delineation of change elements should be provided by a healthcare manager whenever appropriate. How your department reacts to change and positively addresses the characteristics of change should also be discussed. Each member should be given the opportunity to discuss how change will affect his or her particular segment of the business and how the worker might positively address the change at hand. Failing to recognize and communicate change or to identify solutions and strategies toward reacting progressively to change can lead to departmental regression.

Finally, **circumstance** denotes specific conditions under which the department must labor. Conditions might include a change in physical environment, new organization requirements, or regulatory or legislative issues that affect the department. The specific dynamics under which each employee works should also be recognized and discussed, with input garnered from the employee on how best to deal with the particular situations imposed by the job role. Both the morale and overall mission of the department can be bolstered easily and at no cost when the leader **credibly** and **constructively** acknowledges the unique contribution of individual team members.

The Work Community

Any healthcare department is a **unique community**, and it services a community of customers/patients and professionals within the organization who rely on the department to achieve its mission.

The first component of communication as it relates to communal and team orientation is **counsel**. Counsel refers to the ability to provide technical expertise and related needed action throughout the organization. In another sense, counsel refers to the provision of guidance for employees who need specific direction in key areas such as stress management, time management, and family relations. Both you and your human resource department must keep your **counselor** roles at the forefront of strategies when dealing with all members of the organization.

Commitment is dedication to reinforcement of the healthcare mission. All essential organizational messages should be underlined by everyday actions and incorporated in internal communications. This priority of commitment mandates putting the customer/patient at the top and putting service to affiliated members of the organization and to colleagues as a close second priority. Failure to reinforce commitment to the healthcare organizational mission, although a rarity among managers, can occur given everyday hyperactivity of any healthcare organization. Therefore, a savvy healthcare leader will attempt to consciously underscore his organization's commitment to the customer/patient at every opportunity.

The **construction** of a message is very important in community-based communication. In essence, you must know your audience when you construct a message. Some individuals have a high **comprehension** of medical terms; others do not. For the latter group, construction of any message should be based around **concepts** the receiver can easily understand. Messages can sometimes be overloaded, containing information not essential to the desired outcome. In other cases, messages can be too abbreviated and fail to provide essential information. Ensure that your message is well constructed and well measured, given your receiver(s).

Confidence is critically important in delivering any message throughout the healthcare environment. If you lack confidence in what you are saying, you will lose your audience and your credibility. Without credibility, you can be seen as a nonplayer and will have a difficult time gaining respect for your ideas and input. On the other hand, avoid the appearance of being arrogant. Most individuals in the healthcare environment assume you know what you are talking about and that you are capable of making the right decision. There is no reason to **oversell** your ideas, and the risk of doing so is that people will think you are trying **to sell them a bill of goods**.

Because health care is a people-oriented field, a certain amount of **compassion** should be appropriately omnipresent in all your communication efforts. Lack of compassion can suggest that you do not truly care for a patient, a staff member, or whoever is the receiver of your message. However, one can go to extremes in any dimension, so try to avoid being **too compassionate**—that is, considering the humanistic elements in a manner that is disproportionate to the business elements of your objective. However, it is always better to err on the side of being **overly compassionate** than being perceived as not being compassionate enough in a given situation.

Care must be exhibited in everything you do throughout the healthcare community. You should be careful not to offend others needlessly or unwittingly by any communication you provide. Furthermore, patient care should be a driving force in all communication, so ask "How will this communication affect our customers/patients and the quality of care?" Failure to exhibit care in communication can earn you a reputation as being too blunt, brusque, or unfeeling and insensitive toward the needs of others, principally the customer/patient.

Confidence is defined as the net effect of many actions resulting in a increased sense of group competence. A positive **confluence** occurs when several positive factors, such as several departments working **cohesively** together or several employees working toward common goal in a progressive fashion, result in a positive outcome. Conversely, a negative confluence occurs when several negative events produce an overall negative net effect. A strong healthcare organization (and at the department level a strong healthcare team) should seek to create a positive confluence of factors whenever possible. From a communication perspective, this entails continuously identifying and developing positive factors and positive attributes of these factors and pointing them out to all members of your team. As a healthcare manager, you should make this an essential part of your everyday activities.

Any communication process must have **comfort** as an essential dynamic. **The more comfortable someone is, the more he or she will communicate and the more information will emerge.** From an organizational perspective, all individuals should feel comfortable in providing information, giving their opinions, and stating their viewpoints freely and without fear of negative retribution. As a healthcare leader, try to impart these same ideals throughout your department. Strive to maintain a comfortable environment in which you discuss issues with individuals in a nonthreatening manner. By asking questions, you open up **channels** for vital communication; let people know that your office has an air of confidentiality and comfort by closing the door and allowing visitors to sit down and relax while relating problems and situations to you. Without comfort, communication becomes abbreviated and contrived.

Sensitivity to **cultural** diversity is a major management concern. Invariably, you will be challenged with managing culturally diverse individuals along all demographic lines. Cultural conflict can take place in the way individuals communicate. For example, some cultures disapprove of direct eye contact as a sign of disrespect. Other cultures communicate in what may be perceived as a very emotional fashion; others may be perceived as less expressive in their communication style. Recognize these differences objectively, and communicate in a style that is most comfortable for you. Do not try to adopt the cultural norms of others, lest you run the risk of appearing phony or condescending. Communicate in a direct, straightforward manner. Your comfort with your own communication style will be acknowledged by the individuals with whom you communicate and thus will not become a negative issue.

A few guidelines can assist you in making response to cultural diversity a positive attribute of your communication strategy:

- **Never refer to a staff member's cultural background,** even if it is from what you might think is a positive or humorous perspective; you could unknowingly and unintentionally offend the person or make him or her feel uncomfortable.

- **Immediately address any clashes** that might stem from cultural differences among your staff. If allowed to fester, these situations will create immense problems.

- **Do not allow individuals to make cultural differences an issue** in any departmental interchange.

- If ever in doubt or even uncomfortable with a cultural communication or engagement issue, **get an assist immediately** from someone in human resources or senior management.

- If any staff member focuses on using cultural difference as a stumbling block in working with others, **consult your human resource department** as well as your supervisor to resolve this conflict positively and quickly.

Finally, **contact** is essential in community-based communication. The more contact you have with your employees, the more knowledge you will attain about their activities and aspirations. The more contact you have with customers/patients, the greater your knowledge will be of their expectations of the organization and, specifically, their expectations of your department. The more contact you have with your superiors in the organization, the more you will learn about leadership and organizational norms. Finally, the more contact individuals have with you, the more comfortable they will be with relating their ideas and options to you and recognizing you as a leader within the management team.

The Content of Messages

Communicate content involves not only what is said or written but the way in which information is delivered. The best way to examine your proficiency at communication content is to review the following questions and assess your style. Use these 10 components as guidelines for analyzing all your communication activities:

1. **Core:** What is the root of the message? How direct is the message? Is it delivered clearly, understood easily, and capable of being acted on by the receiver?

2. **Clarity:** Is the message clear in intent and purpose? What are its basic elements? What action must be undertaken to support this message?

3. **Comprehensiveness:** What is the full scope of the message? Does it provide all information needed for the desired outcome?

4. **Conciseness:** Did I get to the point? What is the main point of my message? Did I get to the point quickly, without enough foundation? Am I taking too long to get to the point?

5. **Cleverness:** Am I using an appropriate **hook** to get attention? Am I being too **gimmicky** in delivering this message? Could I be more creative in delivering this message?

6. **Character:** Does this message support the basic mission of the organization? Does this message seem consistent with other activities in my department? Does this message relate to something that ultimately will better serve our customers/patients?

7. **Credibility:** How believable is this message? Do I have enough credibility to garner support on the basis of this message? What things should I detail to get the receiver to **buy in** to this message?

8. **Conviction:** Am I stressing the importance of this message enough? Am I displaying how much I believe in the action this message will generate?

9. **Ability to compel:** What action am I asking for? Am I providing enough direction on how to support this message? Am I specifying the time, money, and other quantitative elements of this message strongly enough?

10. **Consequence:** What is the desired outcome of this message? What positive consequences will be realized if this message is followed through? What are some secondary effects of this message? What impact does this message have on the receiver and other individuals in the department?

From a general perspective, it is essential to review all of these C-guidelines prior to delivering your message. As this chapter progresses, more specific message dynamics will be discussed relative to group communication and communication with your supervisor. However, if you follow this guide in all of your management communications, the likelihood of misunderstanding and inaction will be diminished.

The Challenge Communicated by Message

The final category of communication dynamics has to do with **challenge**. It is vital for employees to be challenged and to challenge themselves continuously to become better performers. From a wider perspective, the department must challenge itself to improve performance and to grow and prosper. These final 10 components help contribute to the challenge element of communication:

1. **Comparison:** What positive factors can I compare this action to? What ideals does this action help contribute to? How does this action measure up to our prior successes?

2. **Contrast:** What negative factors can I contrast this message against? What past failures can I contrast it against? What pitfalls will we avoid by following this action?

3. **Closure:** Are we **closing any loops** with this action? What are the logical outcomes of this action? What is a strong finish for this message?

4. **Choice:** What are our options? Is the option in the message our best option? What other choices do I have in order to achieve the desired outcome?

5. **Contract:** What action am I asking for from my staff? What action will I undertake to support this action? What is the mutual benefit of all individual talents in this action?

6. **Customization:** What are some particular dynamics of this action? How does it specifically fit in with our plans? How do I take advantage of all individual talents in this action?

7. **Count:** What are some significant numbers of this action? What are our numerical goals? What are some significant interim numbers?

8. **Cash:** What funds will be saved or generated by this action? What are our budget standards? How can we eliminate revenue waste and operating expenses by this action?

9. **Clock:** What overall time parameters are established by this message? What are the deadlines? How can we eliminate time wasters in pursuing this action?

10. **Clout:** Do we have the authority to take this action? Who should be empowered with the responsibility for this action? Have I been charged with the responsibility and authority to make this happen?

By reviewing these parameters and adhering to these guidelines, you will ensure that motivation and inspiration are a part of all your work-directive communication. Furthermore, by asking yourself these questions, you are ensuring that the pending action is worthwhile and has been fully considered from a totally progressive viewpoint.

Remember, all of these dynamics relate not only to communication style but also to actual delivery of a message. As shown in Figure 10–1, the basic relationship between the sender and the receiver in any communication is vulnerable to obstruction and interference and must be reinforced by the C-Factors discussed in this and preceding subsections. Figure 10–1 shows a number of areas in which communication might be hampered. **How** a message is delivered is always as important as the message itself to the receiver of the message. Therefore, embrace these guidelines as part of your communication strategy in all of your management responsibilities.

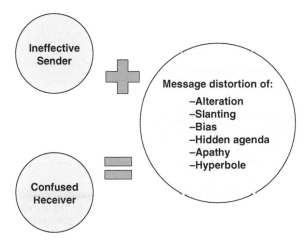

FIGURE 10–1.   Communication distortion.

UNDERSCORING MUTUAL BENEFIT

No matter what psychological playacting or communication tactic an individual might use in a given situation, underscore the mutual benefit of an action as the best tactic for garnering the appropriate response. There are generally 5 recipients of the mutual benefit:

1. The message sender
2. The message receiver
3. The team/staff
4. The organization
5. The customer/patient

Try to identify the individual and operational benefits of an action simply by asking "What are the benefits to each of these parties and to each facet of the business?" Some possible answers (or **payoffs**) are:

Greater effectiveness

Increased efficiency

New programs or evidence of organization progress

Short-term production gains

Long-term positive gains

Staff growth and development

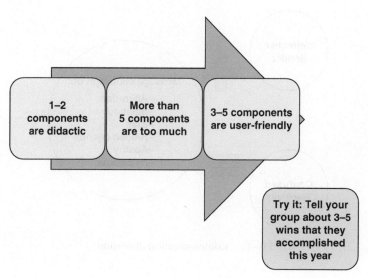

FIGURE 10–2. The 3- to 5-rule of messaging.

By articulating the potential payoffs, you lend maximum clarity to the communication process and stress the contribution needed from each individual in the department. And as depicted in Figure 10–2, utilizing a three- to five-component progression in all messages helps to optimize the efficiency and effectiveness of any message. If a potential recipient fails to respond to the appeal for mutual benefits, you can logically assume that he or she is not truly interested in the positive success of the organization. Put simply, if an individual cannot respond to helping his or her colleagues and organization, that person probably should not be there.

LISTENING KEYS

There are five general rules to remember as part of the critical listening accountability of your communication strategy which augment the **LET** (**L**isten, **E**valuate, and **T**ake Action) strategy presented earlier in this text in a diagram form:

1. Always **listen attentively and accurately** when provided with any type of information.

2. Try to discern not only what someone says **but why they say it**; discount the roles, which can be a distraction and get to the core of the message effectively.

3. Clarity and comfort are a key to communication. **Be clear** about what you are saying, and **be comfortable** in your confidence in saying it.

4. Communication is a continuous process. **Follow up** with individuals on your staff, and always be ready to ask and answer questions.

5. Recognize that learning about communication is a continuous process. Strive to **learn something new about the communication process each day** and apply it as part of your management strategy.

DEALING WITH THE BIGGEST C-FACTOR—CHANGE

With the massive amount of change in the healthcare business arena, both societally and professionally, healthcare managers have been contending with the change management process. Although a breadth of concepts borrowed from other industries and a plethora of conceptual notions have entered the healthcare educational realm, a straightforward, immediately useful approach to managing change is probably more beneficial, as the need to manage change quickly and effectively becomes the paramount criterion for healthcare management success in this decade of change.

In this section, we will explore the areas where mistakes are made most frequently by leaders in the change process, and we will provide specific strategies to not only avoid these mistakes but moreover reduce resistance to change, activate positive action, and ultimately improve performance through optimum staff contribution. The critical areas we will explore are the reasons for resistance to change, the management of the proactive phase of change, creating staff interdependence, and key leadership roles for change management.

There are several prominent group emotions that are triggered by change. These can pervade an entire healthcare team and cause a group counteraction resisting proposed change. The healthcare leader must understand these emotions, their potential deleterious impact, and most importantly, the pragmatic approaches required to manage these emotions toward progressive change. Additionally, the healthcare leader must be aware of the manner in which these emotions specifically affect the 3 performance levels of staff members. These can best be described as the organizational driver or **superstar** level, the **steady** or supporting member level, or the nonplayer **resister** member. The first prominent group emotion usually cited by healthcare leaders as a major factor in the change process is **fear**. As a general sentiment, this factor, as it relates to change, is typified best by the age-old appellation of **fear of the unknown**. However, fear has specific application to healthcare group management, because it can affect all levels of healthcare staff performers in specific manners. For example, the most prominent fear for steady players—who often represent the silent majority of a staff team—is **fear of regression**. Fundamentally, the steady player will view any change with apprehension if the proposed change is not completely presented in a fashion that highlights its improvement value to the status quo. This should be addressed in the proactive phase of change management (as well as see later in this chapter), but as a starting point, the healthcare leader must recognize that most steady staff members will accept change provided it is not simply change for the sake of change. It therefore becomes the responsibility of the leader to identify how the proposed change will bring about new benefits for the customer/patient, the organization, the group, and the individual team member.

The nonplayer staff members are also fearful, but the inspiration for their fear is different, as essentially **the nonplayer fears having to do more work** and change mandates increased effort and higher contribution from all staff members. For steady players and superstars, this requirement is not a problem if it is tied to increased organizational effectiveness and other benefits. For nonplayers, the increased demand for performance is ultimately threatening, because their current level of nonperformance and resistant behavior logically will be exacerbated by more pressure for optimum performance and an accelerated pace of action. Put bluntly, the need for change presents a vibrant opportunity for the nonperformer's laggardness to be found out; that is, the nonplayers will be exposed as incompetent, noncontributory, and detrimental to the provision of stellar health care. Basically, job descriptions and other substantiating criteria are in place for assessing the nonplayer's performance in general and specifically in terms of change and resultant escalated standards for performance, the change dynamic can be an excellent opportunity to appraise the nonplayer's performance justly as substandard and to provide the genesis of terminating the nonplayer for inferior performance. This strategy is truly **rightsizing the right way**, because the successful healthcare organization can only afford to employ individuals who are motivated, competent, and cognizant of the axiom that the organization is more important in the work scheme than individual proclivities, dissenting opinion, and other **me first** mentalities.

For the superstar staff member, fear of change is specifically calibrated to the dimensions of inconsequential outcomes from a proposed change. This concept is best described as a change action that will result in a prevailing sentiment of **so what?** Superstar performers are instinctive in their ability to understand the consequences of an action, and the opportunity to contribute progressively to providing outstanding health care is a guiding beacon in the daily work life of the superstar. Any change in action that is suspect in the eyes of the superstar is a potential **so what?** implementation which can cause the superstar to question the organization's direction and can discourage the superstar, who possesses a high degree of individual positive motivation. It is vital in this regard for the healthcare leader to weigh any potential change relative to organizational readiness and progressive performance, but moreover to engage the superstar's participation in defining potential benefits, operational improvements, and other positive, differentiated improvements to current status and present operational norms.

Other group emotions are also generated by change but usually can be categorized under the aegis of fear. These group phobias of change can include perception versus reality factors regarding change, loss of control relative to one's own professional destiny, and prevailing communication problems that create voids of leadership and accurate communication as well as an array of other potential problems. These negative precursors to change can be managed best by a healthcare leader employing artful strategies throughout the change process and principally in progressive, purposeful change management as depicted in the following sections.

The Planning Phase

The planning phase of the change process is the time before the change dynamic takes place. In this period, the healthcare leader is making plans and motivating staff participation in making the change happen. Many healthcare leaders make the fundamental mistake of entering the change process without proper planning and staff support enlistment. A more progressive approach is to set a course for change and enter a process of garnering staff support by proactively defining the benefits of the imminent change.

The first objective of the planning phase should therefore be a complete delineation of the emergent benefits of the proposed project or new process leading to change. A staff discussion should be led by the manager with the active participation of the superstars and steady players in which all benefits, both apparent and underlying, are identified and related to the change process. Obvious benefits could include more expedient customer/patient service, improved operational flow, or obvious cost savings in relation to operating budget dollars.

Less apparent benefits can also be identified by the group with active leadership from the facilitating manager and the leaders from the staff groups of steady and superstar players. These benefits can include time saved by implementing a new process, energy saved by a more efficient process, lessons that will be learned and technological insight that will be realized by a change in procedure, and any competitive edge that might be afforded by the organization by implementing the change. Underlying benefits can also include better perceptional presence for the department or organization as it embraces a new, vanguard process or a new procedural practice that enables greater accuracy of results, a safer working environment, or a more efficient route to results realization. From an overall perspective, any change that reduces the boredom of a skilled individual, adds to organizational progress (which helps to ensure organizational stability and individual job security), or simply eliminates hurdles or the headaches associated with outmoded or cumbersome processes is one that possesses credible underlying benefit. By eliciting these nonapparent benefits with the group, the healthcare leader adds a flavor of veracity and realism to the change management discussion.

It is essential to completely delineate the plan of change in a **real-world** fashion as the second segment of the planning phase. The manager can construct his or her plan of action by simply answering the following questions:

1. **Why** the change plan must take place, using the benefits identified by the group as the major catalysts
2. **When** the major events in the change plan will occur, using a time sequence of the start, midpoint, and **finished product** elements
3. **How** the plan will take shape, including a visualization of the steps needed to implement the change
4. **Who** will make the plan happen, including an appropriate discussion of group and individual responsibilities

Inherent to this discussion is the necessity of discussing the meaning of the plans. Basically, this discussion of meaning should take two semblance. First, the leader and the group should discuss what the change dynamic will mean in the short term relative to potential implementation problems, variations in daily routine, and any other pertinent topics. Second, the long-term meaning of the change should be discussed fully, replete with a reiteration of benefits, relevance to the big picture of the organization and its relationship with its patient constituency, and other prevailing positive likelihoods. **Too often, the change management discussion focuses only on the short-term pain and not on the long-term gain. Both components must be considered** and especially examined sequentially, so that all members of the group recognize that the initial discomfort will ultimately lead to a better way of doing things.

The third step of the planning phase is the proper management of the communication segment of leadership, particularly regarding the nefarious behavior of the nonplayers. Regardless of the consulting experience of the author, despite the timely use of the first two steps of the planning phase, the nonplayers will use an assortment of verbal contentious challenges to derail the change process. We discussed their general proclivity toward derailment in a previous chapter and now refrain some **counterstrategies** which can help a healthcare leader to achieve sound communication management during the change process particularly in the planning stage when the dissenting nonplayers will take their best shot at negating the positive action of change.

Nonplayer's ploy 1: "That will never work!"

Leader's rejoinder: "Tell us specifically what will work."

Nonplayer's ploy 2: "I have got a problem with this."

Leader's rejoinder: "Redefining problems is useless. Give us a solution that might be useful to achieve our goals."

Nonplayer's ploy 3: "We tried that before, but it did not work."

Leader's rejoinder: "How will this work now, because we are dealing with the present."

Nonplayer's ploy 4: "With all this change, maybe I should find another job."

Leader's rejoinder: "I will accept your resignation immediately, because change will be constant for years to come in health care."

As these techniques indicate, the leader must use three principles in managing the nonplayer's resistance. First, a direct, tactful challenge must be issued to the complaining nonplayer. Under no circumstance should the nonplayer be allowed to simply complain or cast dispersions on group plans without contributing a better idea. The only individual more detrimental to a healthcare organization than a nonplayer in this regard is the manager who allows negativity to become acceptable behavior without holding the nonplayer accountable for constructive contribution, not just their notion of **constructive criticism**—which in their case is really just deliberate and nefarious obfuscation. Second, the leader must use plural pronouns like **we** and **us** so that the entire group recognizes that the nonplayer is questioning the entire group's capability, not just the leader. This encourages the steadies and superstar members to become accountable for group direction and goal formation and enlists their participation in countering ill-conceived negativity. Finally, the leader should use **bottom-line** vernacular, such as **useless** and **immediately**, so that the nonplayers are clear in their understanding that game playing, dissention, and group dedication are intolerable attributes when striving for group achievement.

The final component of the planning stage is the display of natural emotionalism by the group leader. It is imperative that the leader is not phony in displaying a disingenuous **rah-rah** unwarranted positive outlook in the change process. If the leader portrays honest emotion along the appropriate lines suggested in Figure 10–3, the group can readily recognize that the leader is in the same boat as them and continue to row accordingly.

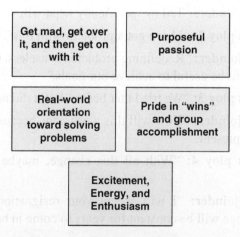

FIGURE 10–3.   Credible leadership emotionalism.

Creating Interdependence

Interdependence among all members of the group is essential to achieving change successfully. Ten basic guidelines must be adhered to if the leader wants all members of the group to reach the implemented change result in a cohesive, integral manner that will provide a sound foundation for future action. These 10 guidelines, presented in a checklist fashion for easy reference, should be used by the healthcare leader as the change process moves from the planning phase to the action phase of the plan:

1. **Identify problems promptly and pragmatically.** This mandates a timely response to cited problems, a practical approach to gathering potential solutions from each staff member, and emphasis on defining new solutions, not reiterating old problems.

2. **Elicit solutions from staff members.** This must be done constantly by consistently asking all group members the question, "How can we do this better?"

3. **Use interactive feedback.** Present critical information to the group on a timely basis, acknowledge and use suggestive feedback, and reward any new innovations that contribute to the process, especially from steady players, using group recognition and other appropriate methods of reward.

4. **Resolve short-term problems and focus on the long term.** Resolve short-term problems quickly by putting the onus for a solution on the individuals identifying the problem first and then charging the group with responsibility of devising a solution that will help make the long-term objective of the change a reality.

5. **Reinforce the need for change.** This should be done throughout the process by asking for new benefits that the change might generate. These benefits would be any advantages the organization, department, or individual might realize that were not identified initially in the planning stage but are now readily apparent and tangible for group identification and discussion.

6. **Cite examples of positive change.** Using the past as a precedent, the leader must make a linkage between past examples of positive group change and current challenges. In fact, most healthcare managers can easily identify a past action that was so daunting that by comparison a current change project is seemingly easy.

7. **Manage the nonplayers strongly and resolutely.** Confronting the nonplayers throughout the process relative to their negativity is the

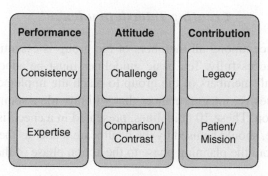

FIGURE 10–4. Thank You to the Fourth Power and reinforcement keys.

responsibility of the leader and should be done using the pronouns **we** and **us** and telling the nonplayers to **stop it or drop it** relative to their negative critique of group movement; that is, unless they can cite a better way, their condemnation of change movement is indeed useless to the group.

8. **Encourage steadies.** Compliment any contribution made by the steadies, highlight their constructive innovations, and commend their performance in public at any juncture to ensure that the silent majority is truly the driving engine of the group change achievement.

9. **Highlight steadies and superstars.** We must all remember in health care that to inspire dedicated performance, time must be taken to say **thank you** (as indicated in Figure 10-4) and to celebrate the wins, not just lament the losses and things that do not go right. The steadies and superstars, as personifications of the goodness of our profession, should be the recipients of positive reinforcement in its most basic form during change specifically and throughout their work life in general.

10. **Use comparison/contrast illustration extensively.** This includes creative use of timelines that shows a before-and-after depiction of the change process or an account of progress made **to date** relative to the change process.

LEADERSHIP ROLES FOR THE CHANGE PROCESS

The essential leadership roles for a healthcare manager to fulfill during the change management role are generally depicted in Figure 10–5. These are eminently familiar to anyone acquainted with popular, established

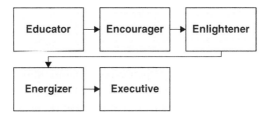

FIGURE 10–5.   Leadership roles in change management.

leadership and management lexicon, and this figure can act as a reflective matrix for the healthcare leader during the change process. However, some of the roles are contained in this merit-specific discussion.

The healthcare manager must be both listener and perceiver throughout the change management process. The distinction between the two roles in this usage would be that a listener understands what a staff member is saying clearly and comprehensively, and a perceiver also understands why someone is making a statement. Understanding the motive behind communication is a leadership responsibility, because communication is a key to action in healthcare performance. The healthcare leader should directly ask a staff member the interrogative, "Why are you telling me this?" to accurately ascertain the need for action and specific response desired by the staff member.

The leader must be an encourager—not just a cheerleader—throughout the change process and fulfill every variation of this role. The leader should be forthright and resolute in displaying the courage necessary to confront, manage, and ultimately redirect or remove nonplayers. This is related to the role of a leader as a coach. This often-used analogy is best considered in this semblance when comparing the need of an athletic coach to motivate 40 different players in 40 different ways. Encouraging leaders must likewise know their players and their specific sources of inspiration and motivation and use this frame of reference pragmatically throughout the change process.

Finally, the leader must be an advocate of three related performance values. First, the leader must always advocate **the need for positivity** to all staff members in an enlightened manner, using strategies we have suggested throughout this article. Second, leaders must advocate **the needs of their staff** in discussions with organizational executives to obtain the necessary resources and support for change process accomplishment. Third, the healthcare leaders must advocate **the position of the entire plurality of the group versus individual concern**, especially those of the low-performance, high-maintenance nonplayers.

SUMMARY

All of us in the medical and healthcare professions know that change is an ever-present reality. It is also a positive motivator for most of us, as it is for the steadies and superstars of our staffs. By focusing our efforts on maximizing their progressive participation in the change process, we can ensure that our vital mission of providing stellar health care to our constituency will be met in the challenging times ahead. This chapter has reviewed an assortment of communication situations and strategies that support the premise that communication is the key to action. By recognizing your communication abilities and constantly developing them, you are in turn constantly developing yourself and growing as a healthcare leader, as good communication and sound leadership and solid management are synonymous. Neither is an exact science, yet both can be attained through constant practice and continual development.

PRACTICAL RESOURCE—CHAPTER X:
The Leader's Guide to Framing a Message

This resource can be used to prepare a presentation to your staff, peers, or reporting executives. It has the **15** important tenets of presentational effectiveness; you need to only follow the prompts of this practical checklist and consider each constructively to fully develop an effective group communication presentation.

Strategic Communication & Leadership Keys

1. **Imagery/Symbols:**
   a. Good pictures
   b. Resonant symbols and iconography
   c. Right mix of graphics and smartart

2. **Visualization:**
   a. Ask the audience to "Picture This"
   b. Relevant scenarios
   c. Present contrasts and comparisons to the status quo

3. **Clarity:**
   a. Keep it simple
   b. Don't be "Too cute by half"
   c. Honest, direct, and thoughtful style

4. **Narration/"The Story":**
   a. Tell an illustrative story
   b. Teach by leading with a story
   c. Ask for an example or exemplar that will tell the story

5. **Product identification:**
   a. Main features of a new service
   b. Main new changes in programs
   c. Launch of new initiatives

6. **Know your customer:**
   a. Primary audience
   b. Secondary audience
   c. Word of mouth generation possibilities

7. **Affiliation links:**
   a. What other departments are involved
   b. What other hospitals are involved
   c. What customer/patient community entities are constituents of this program or project

8. **User-friendly:**
   a. Accessible information
   b. Relevant
   c. Resonant

9. **Aegis/over-arching needs for action:**
   a. Business dimensions
   b. Care imperatives
   c. People management and staffing support

10. **Centric focus:**
    a. What you expect
    b. What your team should expect
    c. What the patient will get

11. **Defining terms:**
    a. Key words
    b. Important argot, parlance, and lexicon
    c. Coin of the realm acronyms

12. **Significant events:**
    a. Major impact events
    b. Historical precedence
    c. External and internal lore, legends, and legacy

13. Critical contributions:
   a. Group supporting action
   b. Your leadership in the process
   c. Organizational resources

14. Call to action:
   a. What you want your audience to do
   b. What you need your organization and team to do
   c. What you would really like to see happen

15. Starting point(s):
   a. "Here's how I'm going to get this started"
   b. "Here's how you (the listener) can get involved"
   c. "Here's who else/what we need for this to start happening"

Index